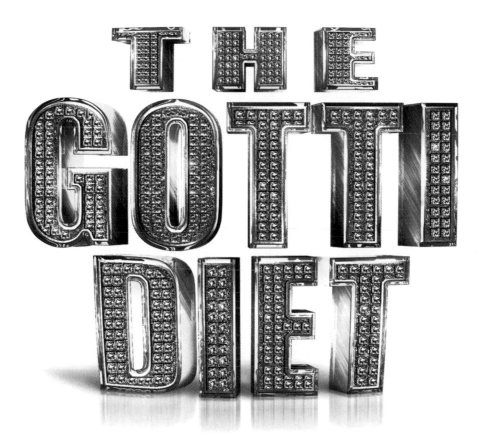

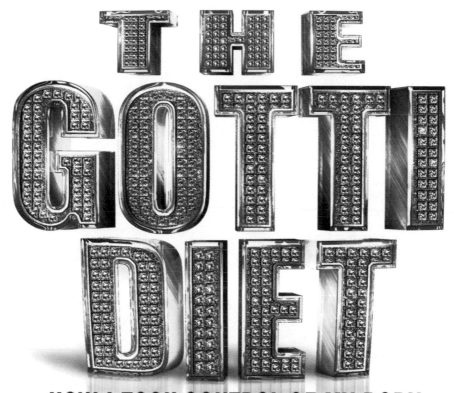

THE GOTTI DIET

HOW I TOOK CONTROL OF MY BODY
LOST 80 POUNDS
AND DISCOVERED HOW TO STAY FIT FOREVER

Frank Gotti Agnello

Costar of the hit A&E series *Growing Up Gotti*

10 ReganBooks
Celebrating Ten Bestselling Years
An Imprint of HarperCollinsPublishers

This book contains advice and information relating to health care. It is not intended to replace medical advice and should be used to supplement rather than replace regular care by your doctor. It is recommended that you seek your physician's advice before embarking on any medical program or treatment. All efforts have been made to assure the accuracy of the information contained in this book as of the date of publication. The publisher and the author disclaim liability for any medical outcomes that may occur as a result of applying the methods suggested in this book.

PHOTOGRAPHY CREDITS: All exercise photographs in Chapter 7 by Quentin Bacon. All other photographs courtesy of the author.

HarperCollins books may be purchased for educational, business, or sales promotional use. For information please write: Special Markets Department, HarperCollins Publishers Inc., 10 East 53rd Street, New York, NY 10022.

FIRST EDITION

Designed by Kris Tobiassen
Hand lettering by AKA Studios and Michelle Ishay

Printed on acid-free paper

Library of Congress Cataloging-in-Publication Data has been applied for.

ISBN 0-06-083289-4

05 06 07 08 09 RRD 10 9 8 7 6 5 4 3 2 1

TO MY MOTHER AND FATHER

**All my thanks for raising me, loving me, and helping me
stick to my diet and fitness plan.**

CONTENTS

INTRODUCTION
Why I'm Writing This Book ix

IT'S NO FUN TO BE FAT
STEP 1: Acknowledge You've Got a Weight Problem 1

YOU CAN'T WALK ALONE
STEP 2: Ask for Help . . . and Ask for Support 19

IT'S BETTER THAN A GOOD IDEA
STEP 3: Make the Mind-Body Connection 25

CIAO CHOW
STEP 4: Examine Your Eating Habits: The What, When, Where, and Why 31

MANGIA! MANGIA!

STEP 5: Learn to Make Better Food Choices 63

GET MOVING!

STEP 6: Get to the Heart of Weight Loss with Exercise 77

EXERCISES I DO TO STAY FIT

STEP 7: Lift Extra Pounds, Don't Gain Them 93

TRACKING YOUR OWN SUCCESS

Recording Your Weight-Loss, Food, and Fitness Plan 115

I CAN DO ANYTHING

The Proof Is in My Body! 135

A MOTHER'S UNCONDITIONAL LOVE

My Mom Has Something to Say 143

RECIPES FOR SUCCESSFUL WEIGHT LOSS

Tasty Foods That Satisfy Your Appetite 151

Glossary 207

Acknowledgments 217

INTRODUCTION
WHY I'M WRITING THIS BOOK

"Teenagers in the United States have higher rates of obesity than those in fourteen other industrialized countries, including France and Germany, a study of nearly thirty-thousand youngsters ages thirteen and fifteen found.

"Among American fifteen-year-olds, fifteen percent of girls and nearly fourteen percent of boys were obese, and thirty-one percent of girls and twenty-eight percent of boys were more modestly overweight."

I heard this on CNN, so it *has* to be true. And, if I hadn't come to grips with my own weight issues, I would have proven these statistics to be true.

From the time I was six years old until I turned thirteen, I was a fat kid. By the time I started school, there was no way to rationalize my weight as "baby fat." When

I had my seventh-grade physical for school, I weighed 255 pounds, up from the 236 I weighed the previous summer. That wouldn't have been such a bad weight if I were as tall as Shaquille O'Neal, but I wasn't. I was just under six feet—five-ten-and-a-half—to be exact. Two hundred-fifty-five is at least seventy pounds too many for a guy my height and build.

I didn't start out fat—when I was born I weighed seven pounds, or less. (Either my brother John or I weighed seven pounds and the other, six pounds, fourteen ounces. Mom can't remember which.)

I wasn't even a chubby little boy when I was in kindergarten, but by the time

When I made my first Communion, I was eight years old and weighed more than both of my older brothers.

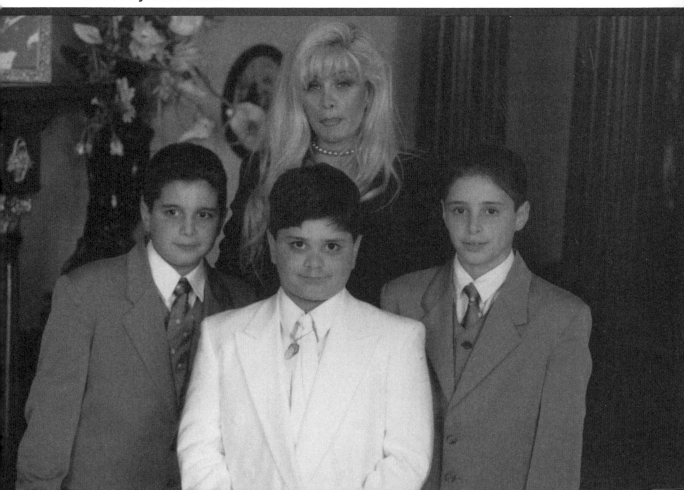

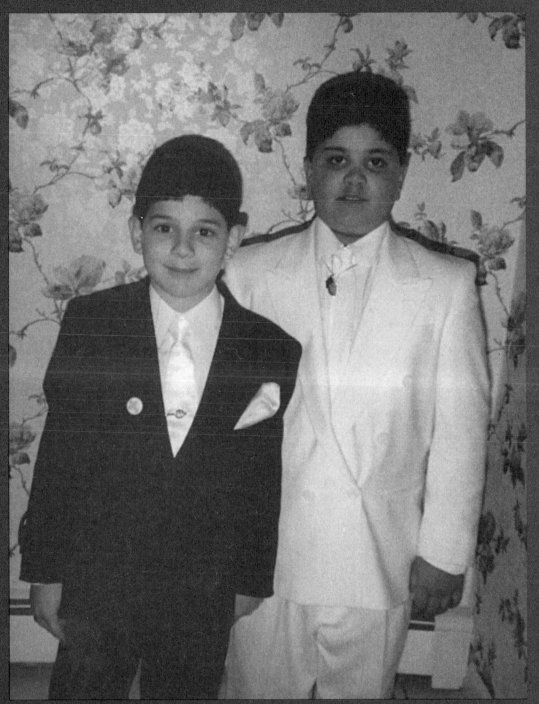

My cousin Frank and I were both named after our uncle who died when he was a kid; we were born two months apart, and we grew up side by side. By the time we were eight, I was already half a head taller and many pounds heavier than he.

I turned six, I had started packing on the pounds. I had a moon face and pudgy body. I was round. Nobody paid much attention to how much I ate—after all, growing boys are expected to be "good eaters." My, what a good appetite I had.

And, since I'm from a big Italian American family that truly appreciates a good meal, there was always plenty of food on the table for me to eat. And so I did. Mom even taught me how to cook some of our favorite dishes, so I could help out.

Between meals, there were plenty of snacks for me to grab, too—ice cream, soda, candy, cookies—and I enjoyed them all, especially the ice cream. For a while there, I ate a pint of the stuff in one sitting—Rocky Road . . . or anything else chocolate—straight from the container. If Häagen Dazs, Baskin-Robbins, and Cold Stone Creamery gave frequent flyer miles, I would have been able to go around the world a couple of times.

I don't know that I ate much more than my brothers did when they were six and seven or so, but I must have. While Carmine and John had grown lean and wiry, I got fat, and I kept getting fatter.

I'm lucky. Unlike lots of fat kids, my classmates didn't make fun of me, calling me names like Fat Boy, Fatso, and Lard Ass. I've heard about guys who hated going into the lunchroom at school because, no matter what they were eating, somebody had something nasty to say about it: "Look at the Pig!" or "Hey Fat Ass! Are you sure you're really going to eat that?"

I wasn't totally free of ridicule. Although my brothers would try to tease me at home, my mother wouldn't allow any of it.

When I decided to change my life, I was fat, *very* fat. It was clear to me that I had to get a grip on my weight. Clearly, I would have to alter what I ate and start an exercise program. As if I needed any added kick in the pants to get started, talk of our family doing a reality TV show that would be called *Growing Up Gotti* was beginning to move from being a good idea into a strong possibility.

I was determined to lose the excess weight I had been hauling around for as long as I could remember, especially if there was going to be a TV camera following me around once *Growing Up Gotti* went into production. I didn't want to be known as "Fat Frankie" throughout the entire country.

I knew I could lose the weight; I just didn't know how I would do it. The first hurdle I had to jump over was discovering how I would eat less to lose weight. I suppose I knew, deep down, that I had been eating too much. But I had been turning to food as a source of comfort for so long I had no idea how to stop.

As for exercise, the story was the same. I had phys-ed classes and played basketball and lacrosse at school, but I had rarely done any other regular, *legitimate* physical activity since I played Little League baseball. I often played in pickup games in our backyard with my brothers and friends, but most of the time, I have to admit, I was extremely lazy. I just sat around in front of the TV or my computer screen and snacked on whatever was there for the eating.

To tell the truth, when I was fat, I really couldn't run far. In fact, I hated to run because I couldn't go for more than a minute before I started breathing extremely heavily and feeling like I was going to collapse.

A lot has been said about being overweight or eating disorders with girls in mind. Everybody knows about some super-skinny actress or model who goes off to rehab for treatment of anorexia or some other eating disorder or the supersized singer who gets her stomach stapled. However, as I started boning up on what I needed to do to get in shape, I couldn't understand why, but I couldn't find a thing that talked specifically about overweight boys. That was odd because I knew I wasn't the only fat boy in the world. I mean, I wasn't even the only fat boy in my school.

Maybe the weight issues of girls are more obvious than with guys. Look at the very thin models and celebrities pictured in magazines and gossiped about on TV. I've heard girls talking about what star had an eating disorder, who followed what diet, and which were the best exercises to do.

But for us guys, what are we supposed to do? Tough it out? Nobody's talking about it, but fat boys suffer too, don't we? You'll never hear a guy ask a buddy, "Hey man, do you think these jeans make my butt look fat?" We just don't talk about it.

That was about the time I knuckled down and waged my own campaign on my weight. In barely a year's time, I have grown two inches, to six-feet-one-inch tall, and, most importantly, I have lost almost eighty pounds. I watch what and how much I eat, and I work out, even if it's just a little bit, every day. Now I keep free weights—dumbbells—in my room, so I can do lifts and presses while doing my homework or watching TV. It keeps me busy, and, when I was just starting my diet, it kept my mind off eating.

At first, friends and family members teased me about my new eating habits. They weren't supportive. They even said they doubted if I'd be able to stick to my plan. They figured I'd get bored after a couple of months, or at least hungry, and give up my crusade after a few weeks—six weeks tops. Thanks guys.

Now they admit that they've seen the results of my diet and exercise program and tell me that I've even inspired other people to lose weight and get in shape. While Carmine and John used to kid me about being too fat, now they razz me about being too skinny. A couple of months ago, when we were starting to shoot season two of *Growing Up Gotti,* John was telling me that my bones are showing . . . and that I should gain some weight. That won't happen. Not since I've gone from fat to fit.

When my cousin Bobby came to me and said he wanted help to lose weight, I felt like, for once, *I* was a role model. It was kind of hard to believe but cool at the same time. I felt proud, but I told him that if he really wanted my help, he had to know right up front that I wasn't going to kid around with him and let him cheat.

Bobby told me, "You know Frank, I see how you refuse to eat Wendy's and all that. I don't want to eat that way any more either. I'm going on a diet. Help me out."

Within the first three weeks he had lost about nine pounds, but, one day, when he and his mom Susan walked into our house, Susan said to me, "I'm not going to lie to you, Frankie, but on the way here, Bobby told me to stop at a McDonald's, so he could eat before he came here."

Since his mom didn't stop, Bobby got over that hurdle. Hey, I never promised losing weight would be easy.

Bobby isn't the only one who has asked for my help. Other kids my age have contacted our *Growing Up Gotti* website, asking for tips on how to get started and what they need to do to lose weight and get fit.

I swear I don't have any special powers, just my intense desire to get in shape. I'm stubborn and tired of being teased, taunted, and being made the butt of people's jokes. I was fed up with feeling sluggish and awkward. I couldn't wear some of the cool clothes that looked so good on Carmine and John. I was the slob in baggy sweats who didn't look like he cared a bit about his appearance. But I did care—and I was trying to hide what I really looked like from everyone.

So I summoned up the will to handle my weight before it got the best of me. The result of my quest to get fit can be summed up in these seven steps:

STEP 1: Acknowledge you've got a weight problem

STEP 2: Ask for help . . . and ask for support

STEP 3: Make the mind-body connection

STEP 4: Examine your eating habits

STEP 5: Learn to make better food choices

STEP 6: Get to the heart of weight loss with exercise

STEP 7: Lift extra pounds, don't gain them

This 7-step program is the result of my own yearlong quest to go from fat to fit. I share it with you to inspire you to do what *you* have to reach your own ideal weight and level of fitness. I'm living proof that it's possible—and it works.

I won't promise that you'll lose seventy-five or eighty pounds in a year and a half like I have, but I can say that by stepping up to the plate and taking a swing at your well-being, you will begin to feel better about yourself and your body. The better you feel about your body, the easier it will be to stick to your get-fit plan.

Ask your parents to take you in for a physical, and let your doctor know what you intend to do. Who knows, he or she may have some ideas specifically about what you need to do for your own body.

And, if your family and friends aren't completely supportive of your efforts to lose weight and get fit in the beginning, ignore them! Your decision to get fit and healthy may be one of the most important tasks you ever tackle.

Do this, and you can do anything you set your mind to.

—FRANK GOTTI AGNELLO

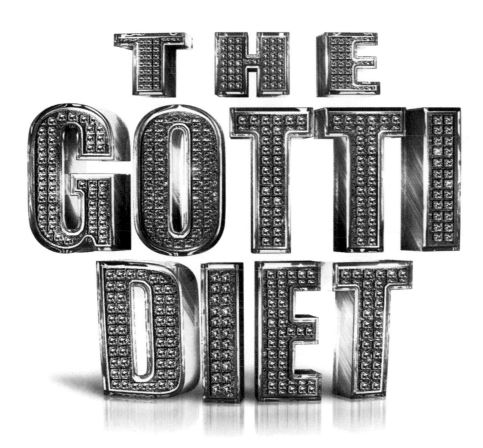

IT'S NO FUN TO BE FAT

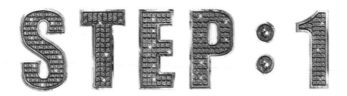

STEP:1

ACKNOWLEDGE YOU'VE GOT A WEIGHT PROBLEM

I got fat all by myself. I didn't get that way overnight, and I certainly didn't do it on purpose. I was a kid; I was *growing;* I ate . . . and I got fat. That's how it happens, isn't it?

I wasn't the only one, but I certainly was the biggest (translation: fattest) kid in my class all through grade school.

In the lunchroom, I was self-conscious. I didn't want to hear anyone say things like "Hey Fat Frankie! Whatcha eating now?"—like I wasn't supposed to get hungry or eat lunch.

At recess, I was self-conscious too. I was pretty active, but because I was larger and clumsier than everyone else I was often the last one picked for team. It didn't

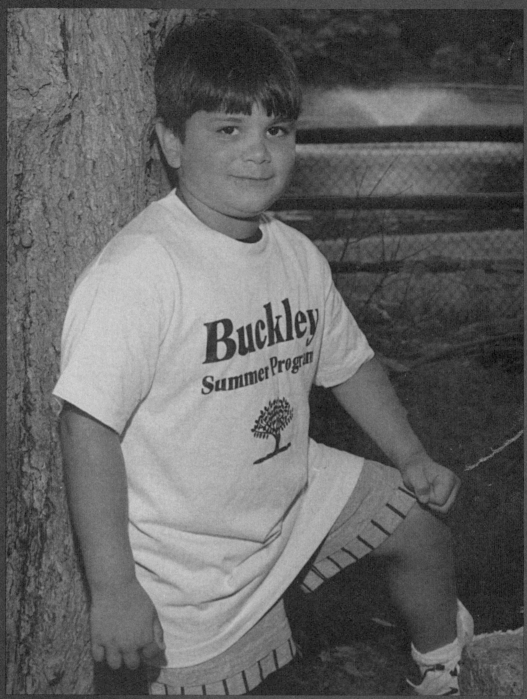

I was the largest second grade kid around the summer I went to Camp Buckley. This didn't stop me from running around, swimming, or anything else, though I didn't know I was already on the road to getting really fat.

matter that I was pretty good at basketball and lacrosse; my size made people think that, because I was fat, I wasn't good at sports.

When my brothers and I went to the same school, Carmine and John ran interference for me, even if they didn't actually do anything. They let me fight my own battles. My brothers also knew I could take care of myself if I really had to.

This is not to say that Carmine and John didn't give me a hard time when Mom wasn't looking. I think that sometimes they were embarrassed to be seen in public with me, and they teased me—big time. We'd be kidding around, and the next thing you'd know, we'd be in a shoving match, and they'd be hollering names at me: "Get out of here, Fatty. . . . Go eat something, Fatso!"

One time, one of them grabbed a newly opened box of chocolate-covered Entenmann's doughnuts off the kitchen counter and shoved it in my face. "Here! Eat this, Blimp!"

The badgering hurt, but I swallowed my pain and my pride—along with massive quantities of food—like I deserved to be put down. I just went home from school and ate. That was always a safe place for me to eat. Besides, Mom always made sure we had snacks, things to make sandwiches, sodas—anything we might want—when my brothers and I came in from school with our friends, and I took advantage of it all.

I remember that I ate everything in this smorgasbord of after-school treats, but now that I think about it, I don't remember tasting it. I just ate. It was all about quantity, and the more I ate, the less I felt.

And when we had company, I almost always helped serve the food. I was so well-mannered, so generous . . . and so close to the kitchen.

When I went to the beach with friends or when everyone came out to our house to go into the pool, I wouldn't take off my shirt. I would do the normal "fat" thing and go in with a T-shirt on, or I would wait on the side until everyone else had been in the water for 20 minutes or so—so they wouldn't notice me—and then I'd rip off my shirt and jump in. Then, when I was done, I would run to the nearest towel and cover myself up.

Family gatherings weren't much better. I remember hearing grown-ups say, "Frank has such a beautiful, handsome face . . . *tsk, tsk.*" While no one ever came out and actually said anything to my face, I intuitively knew they were avoiding the obvious, the elephant in the living room: my weight.

I spent a lot of time sitting in front of the TV between the ages of nine and ten. Believe it or not, this picture was taken in a hotel room when we were on a family vacation! Why wasn't I out playing on the beach?

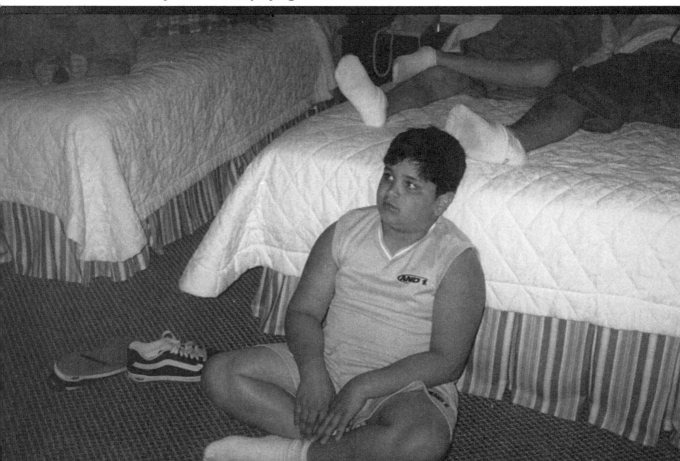

And if anyone had the nerve to ask me how much I weighed, I'd lie and subtract fifteen or twenty pounds from the real number, like it really made a difference.

I never was one of those fat kids who became the class clown or practical joker. And I didn't turn into one of those jerks who would elbow his way through the halls at school or in the mall like he was the juggernaut of a massive army of soldiers either. You know the type—it's as if they're telling the world, "If you think I'm fat, I'll just *show* you how big I am." I didn't do that.

Most of the time I locked myself in my room—my personal space—and mentally beat myself up for being so fat. But all I ever did about it was eat. And this wasn't helped in the least by the fact that my mom and dad had just told me and my brothers that they were getting a divorce.

I was just an eleven-year-old kid, and, as far as I could tell, my family—my whole world—was being ripped apart right around me. I couldn't talk about my feelings with Carmine and John either because they were dealing with the situation themselves, each in his own way.

And, as I saw it, Mom had too much on her mind for me to unload my fears on her, so I couldn't talk to her about things either. Without anyone to talk to, I turned to food to make myself feel better, to numb my fears and feelings.

I imagined all sorts of horrible things, like that we would have to move from the only home I'd ever known. When I was born, we lived in Atlantic Beach, but we moved into this house in Old Westbury that was my mother's dream home before I was two. I was afraid I would have to leave my school and all the friends I had known most of my life, and that I would have to start over someplace else.

From the day Mom filed for divorce, I became more and more frightened, and the more frightened I became, the more I ate. Food became my only pleasure, my only source of security and comfort. The only time I felt secure was when I had a full stomach.

By the time I went into middle school, my weight—and my eating—were completely out of control. I had always been kind of shy and quiet, compared to my brothers, but now, my self-esteem was in the dumps.

The following July, when I went in for my next back-to-school physical, I was twelve years old; I weighed 236 pounds and stood five feet, ten-and-a-half inches tall. I was about the same height as my dad and weighed only about twenty pounds less. Dad needed to lose a few pounds too, but at least he was an adult. Then I heard Dr. Steve Rucker, who's been our family pediatrician for as long as I can remember, tell my mother that I was *morbidly obese*. Talk about scary.

The phrase "morbidly obese" echoed through my head. I was familiar with the word "obese" and, since I knew the word "morbid," I figured that "morbidly obese" meant I was so fat I might die. That really *was* morbid.

Dr. Rucker went on to explain that my blood pressure was 140/90, which, he assured Mom and me, was "dangerously high" for a twelve-year-old. (110/70 or 120/80—that would have been good.) The good news, he said, was that my cholesterol and triglycerides levels were fine, whatever that meant.

Then Dr. Rucker started talking about all the problems I was setting myself up for by being so overweight. While they were in the safe range at that moment, my cholesterol levels could climb, and I would be in danger of getting all sorts of diseases in the future—diabetes, coronary artery disease, stroke . . . joint pain, arthritis, kidney stones, especially if there was a family history. The list went on. I was shocked. Those are diseases that *old* people get! I wasn't just big or fat or overweight any more. I was morbidly obese.

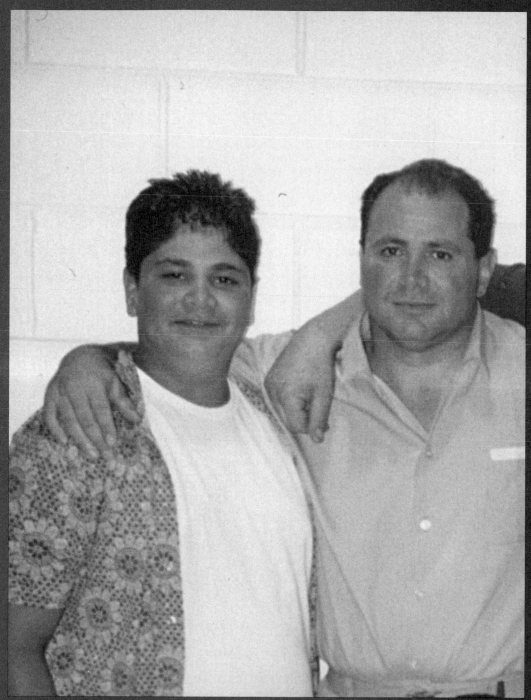

By the time I hit twelve, I was as big as my dad, standing five-feet, ten-and-a-half-inches tall and weighing 236 pounds. When I went for my school physical exam, I found out I had hypertension—high blood pressure—too.

Dr. Rucker talked to Mom and me about my obvious need to lose weight. He even recommended a diet, but it didn't work out. I honestly tried to do what he said, but I couldn't stick to it. Before long I started eating fatty foods again.

Then, for a while, I simply tried to cut back on what I ate. "Cutting back" is a relative thing. I could cut back from two helpings of fettuccine with white clam sauce to one, but what good was that if I put as much food in the bowl for that one serving as I'd eaten when I was going back for refills?

These initial attempts to lose weight were all-out failures. In only a week or two, my fear of being morbidly obese got the better of me. In a panic, I completely lost control. I was eating more than ever.

I went right back to uncontrolled overeating. There were days when I would come home from school and fix myself a sandwich and heat up a can of soup, even though I had already eaten a full lunch at school only a couple of hours earlier. I would eat all of that and then make some more. It was not uncommon for me to have five bowls of soup between school and dinnertime, and then I would sit down and eat a full meal—large, double helpings of everything Mom fixed for dinner. There might be macaroni and cheese, mashed potatoes, spaghetti or lasagna with sauce and cheese, fried chicken cutlets, everything I loved. For me, a single serving of ice cream was the container it came in. And, as I've said, my mom's a great cook.

Between dinner and the time I went to sleep, I ate ice cream—not bowls or servings, but pints. Nothing in our refrigerator was safe.

I knew I needed to get a grip on my eating habits, but I couldn't do it without taking some drastic measures. I was absolutely, completely, out of control.

All that summer, I made a point of exercising. That is, I played ball with my brothers and friends who gathered at our house. I also played a lot of our own version of water polo, which amounted to a raucous round of dodge ball in our back-yard pool. But I ate.

Once, hoping for a quick fix since it was apparent that I wasn't going to be able to stop eating too much, I ordered one those fancy "reducing belts" that supposedly sends electric charges through your abdominal muscles to simulate exercise. I'd seen it advertised on TV, and it sounded good to me. The intensity and rhythm of the contractions supposedly tighten your abs. It felt cool. I actually thought it could work.

When the UPS man delivered this magic belt, my brothers and I started playing around with it. One of us put it around our mom's waist and turned it on. "Hey, Ma, you've gotta feel this!"

This turned out to be a problem. We had failed to realize that the electrical charge in the belt would affect her heart. Our mom has a device implanted in her chest to regulate her heartbeat if it needs it, and the pulsing charge of the belt set off the device.

Mom spent the night in the hospital, and I was overcome with guilt. So I ate.

The next summer, when I went in for my back-to-school check-up, my recorded weight was 255 at the age of thirteen. I was even more morbidly obese than I had been the summer before.

TAKING STEPS ON MY OWN

Finally, I broke down and asked my mom to help me find a diet I could go on, so I could lose weight. She told me she had heard good things about Weight Watchers and rounded up some information about the Weight Watchers food plans.

When we found out that there were no Weight Watchers meetings specifically for kids around where we live, she even offered to go with me. Now, Mom has never had a problem with her weight in her life, but she had seen my aunt and several of her friends struggle to stay slim. She was willing to say that I had come with *her*, since she couldn't get a sitter to stay with me at home, but I said no. Nobody would ever believe *she* was going to a meeting of Weight Watchers.

Mom and I looked into those high protein no-and low-carbohydrates diets like Atkins and the South Beach Diet, but as soon as I was about to start on one of these plans, she found out that, while you can lose a lot of weight in a short amount of time, you also can gain it back very quickly when you start eating bread and pasta again.

I knew that wouldn't work for me. I couldn't imagine spending the rest of my life without pasta.

What I did know for sure was that I had to eat less to lose weight. I also knew that some foods—like fried chicken, mashed potatoes and gravy, macaroni and cheese, cheese and meat ravioli and sauce, ice cream and chocolates—weren't good for me if I was going to lose weight. And I knew that other foods—like lean meats, salads, vegetables and fruits—*were*.

Common sense told me that if I could simply cut down the *quantity* of the food I ate, and, if I ate only the foods that were healthy, I *might* have a shot at losing weight. I also knew that I'd need to get more exercise than I got from gym class and recess to get into shape. I could no longer sit around like a lump in front of the TV. I had to get moving. What could be more logical?

So, in the summer of 2003, I got serious about losing weight. You could say that this was when I took the first step of what is now my *7-Step Program for Successful Weight Loss for Teenagers.*

I was determined to go on a diet that worked for me, and I was committed to be strict about it. I decided that I would try to balance things out. That meant I would balance out my diet and eat a little of everything—proteins *and* carbohydrates—and I would develop a balanced exercise program that would include both aerobic exercise and weight training.

I would explore the world of moderation. For starters, I would eat less—only one helping of everything per meal and no dessert.

This moderate way of eating worked, but I wasn't seeing any rapid results. So I eliminated bread, pasta, and potatoes—starchy foods—from my diet altogether, and I started eating salads—big ones—with a nice piece of steak or grilled chicken: nothing fried; no pasta, potatoes, or bread; no snacks; no ice cream; no chocolate.

And, when my brothers and our friends got on my case and kidded me about how I was eating, I just picked up my plate and went to my room and ate by myself. I didn't have to do that often. I guess they began to get the picture: I meant business. When they weren't going to get a rise out of me, they quit waving desserts and fried foods in my face.

Then I asked my brothers and our friends to keep an eye on me. I said, "If you ever see me going for something bad, like bread, fries, or anything like that, stop me . . . because I'm dead serious about this. I'm going to lose this weight."

They all said, "Yeah, yeah . . . okay Frank. Sure."

The guys really didn't believe I could stick to my guns. In fact, they all laughed about it, but they watched me go through it, waiting for me to fail.

I stuck with it and ate nothing but salads with light dressing and a piece of steak or grilled chicken for lunch and dinner and the occasional piece of fruit. Luckily, my school cafeteria had a salad bar, so I could stick to my program even at school. It wasn't much, mostly greens and raw things, but it was better than meat, potatoes, and the other usual meals they served.

Most often though, I waited until I got home from school and fixed something for myself. That way I had some control over what I was eating. I do know that some people bring a meal replacement shake or bar to eat rather than taking a chance that there'd be nothing on the menu to eat, but as far as I'm concerned these "diet aids" taste too much like candy and milk shakes—some of my very favorite things to eat. Instinct told me I could get myself in trouble if I fed my sweet tooth, even with supposedly "safe" sweets.

I also gave up Coke, Pepsi, and every other kind of soda—even the diet kind—and made certain that I drank plenty of water to wash metabolized fat and wastes from my system. I had read someplace that this was important, so I took it to heart, drinking as much as a gallon of water a day.

And, believe it or not, I didn't go hungry. The water made me feel full and, consequently, cut my appetite.

Before I knew it, the impossible happened: I had lost my taste for soda. I don't even like them any more, which is big, since I used to drink a liter or more a day. In the past couple of months, I've had the occasional bottle of diet iced tea or Diet Coke, but definitely not like I drank soda before!

And I've lost my urge for chocolate. Oh, I may have a chocolate rush once in a while, but I stop myself. I won't eat it. I don't even crave ice cream anymore; I don't want it.

After lunch, I always make a point of going outside to run around, play a little basketball. This is especially important at school, since this activity gets that heavy feeling out of my stomach and gives me energy for the rest of the day.

I have played sports for as long as I can remember—from Little League baseball in grade school to basketball and lacrosse as I got older, but I can honestly say I've never been as active as I am now. Before, mostly, I sat around in front of the TV or hung out in my room doing nothing much at all.

As I lost weight and became stronger, I have had more energy than I can remember. As a result, I am more active. As a result, my body is better able to burn calories, and, since I'm not eating as much as I did a year ago, I'm burning up fat.

I know that helped me lose the weight, and it also helped me firm up and get in shape. Concentrated activity burns calories and that means weight loss, so I increased my exercise and activity level by a lot.

Then, I started working out with weights. We have a bench and weights set up downstairs in our basement, so, at first, I worked out there. This soon got monotonous, so I decided to take some dumbbells up to my room to work out there where I could watch TV and listen to music.

Now, when I get bored or fidgety, I pick up my weights and burn off that nervous energy.

I started doing simple curls and lifts—exercises to tone my biceps, triceps, and pecs—and then I added sit-ups and crunches to tighten my abs. I'll be explaining the basic exercises I do in the chapter entitled "Exercises I Do to Stay Fit," page 93.

And I've started going to a gym where I can work out with a trainer who can teach me what to do to become totally fit and trim.

I know that opinions differ about how old a person should be to start working with weights. That's between you, your parents, your family doctor, and your coach. Obviously, if you are still growing, your body has not matured enough for you to safely incorporate serious weight training into your exercise program. All I can say is that this is the program that has worked for me. It's no frills and basic.

By the time we started shooting our TV show, *Growing Up Gotti,* I felt much better about myself. I hadn't reached my weight-loss goal, but I felt like I looked like a normal kid my age. Talk about a dose of self-confidence.

By the time I went in for my 2004 back-to-school physical, I weighed 178—seventy-seven pounds less than the previous summer. Dr. Rucker didn't even recognize me at first. He was amazed at what I'd been able to accomplish in a year's time, telling my mom and me that he'd never known a kid to be so motivated, especially a guy.

All I can say is that it's no fun to be fat . . . but being fit feels great.

The closest thing to a problem I have with my body now is, believe it or not, stretch marks! Before I lost weight, my skin was stretched. Now, places of my skin looked like the stretched out rubber of a deflated balloon. I could see tiny, silvery, white lines in places where I had been especially fat, under my upper arms especially.

Not long ago, I was changing my shirt, and my mom noticed them. I got really self-conscious, and she picked up on it. "What's the matter?" she asked.

I showed her what was going on with my skin and asked if she knew if there was anything I could do about it.

Mom explained that I had stretch marks, that women usually got them after having a baby. She said she even had them, but that you can't see them anymore. She said she spread cocoa butter on her skin to erase the stretch marks—something called shea butter is good too.

So I'm adding that to the assembly of grooming products I'm using now: deodorant, aftershave, hair gel . . . and cocoa butter.

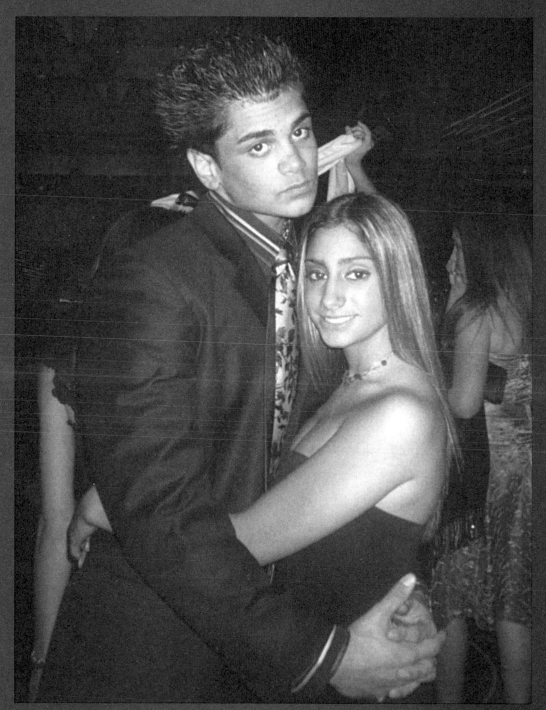

When it was time for the fall social my freshman year, I was ready to go. I felt confident . . . and I felt cool as I danced with my girlfriend, Nikki.

Hey, if that's my only problem, I'm a very lucky guy.

The outgrowth of my yearlong weight-loss and fitness campaign is this 7-step program that I am offering to you now. Use it as a road map to healthy weight loss, and see where it leads you. Read on, and put these steps to work.

Just remember: Losing weight and getting fit is simple, even obvious after you've done it, but not for one minute is it easy.

Are you ready to start on your healthy weight loss program? If you are, it's time to take the first step.

STEP 1: ACKNOWLEDGE YOU'VE GOT A WEIGHT PROBLEM.

After years—for me, it was a lifetime—of being overweight and out of shape, some turning point, some event, may push you over the line. Something will cause you to acknowledge you've got a problem with your weight. It might be that your pecs are so flabby you won't take off your T-shirt at the beach because you *know* someone will laugh at you for having tits. Or you heard a girl you really liked (or, if you're a girl, you heard a guy you really like) tell a friend that your "love handles" made you look like you were standing in the middle of an inner tube. It might even be something to do with your health, like you started having trouble breathing when you had to walk upstairs to history class on the third floor after having lunch on the first floor.

All the teasing from friends and classmates, all the cajoling from parents, all the wishing and hoping in the world is worthless until *you, and you alone*, acknowledge that your weight is a problem.

So, Step 1 is your chance to jump-start you on your way to moving from fat to fit. Your mom and dad can be on your case every day. You can look in the mirror and see how big you are getting; you can step on the scale and watch the numbers rise, and you can hear the names people call you behind your back, but **if you can not openly acknowledge that you have a problem with your weight, you can't *begin* to get it under control.**

Remember, it's not what people say about you or the nasty names they call you. It's what you say about yourself that counts. Ironically, some of us are more hateful to ourselves than we are to perfect strangers. A friend told me about a guy who *oinked* like a pig and shoved his way through a group of boys who made fun of him for being so fat. His self-hatred was every bit as ugly as the actions of his tormenters. The Golden Rule may say we should do unto others as we would have them do unto us. I say we should start out doing unto *ourselves* as we would do unto others.

Practice telling yourself that you deserve to have a fit, healthy body at a suitable weight for your body frame and height. Keep reminding yourself of this until you believe it. Just *wanting* to lose weight and look "normal" won't cut it. You've got to face the problem head-on and take action to get some results.

YOU CAN'T WALK ALONE

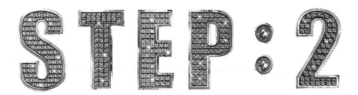

ASK FOR HELP . . . AND ASK FOR SUPPORT

Once you've come to terms with the fact that you have a problem with your weight, you're ready to take Step 2:

STEP 2: ASK FOR HELP

Let the people around you know what you are doing and ask for their support. Your family and friends know you and care about you . . . no matter what you weigh. You may even be surprised to learn that they've been concerned about your weight too, but they didn't know what to say or do about it.

You may even learn a few things about your family, like I did. I came by the tendency to be overweight quite naturally. While on my mother's side—the Gottis—the tendency is to be more lean and muscular than fat, there are those who have had to battle their weight or else they'll get chubby, not obese. My dad's family—the Agnellos—however, is a different story. I don't remember ever seeing my dad thin—he's always been in the 245- to 275-pound range—and there are several relatives who you might say are dangerously obese. In fact, according to Agnello family lore, my dad's cousin Margaret was so fat that her heart just gave out. She spent the last years of her life holed up in her house on Long Island, lying alone in her room, away from the world, doped up on antidepressants and crying her eyes out. Simple errands were out of the question, and, when she had to go out to the doctor, the fire department had to come and cut out the upstairs window to her bedroom just to lift her out of the house and, when she died, she had to be buried in a piano case.

That could have been where I was headed if I hadn't made the decision to get rid of my excess weight.

When I asked friends to speak up if they saw me going for fried foods or anything else they thought I shouldn't be eating if I were going to lose weight, I meant it. At first, they teased me big time, but once they realized how serious I was about getting in shape, they came around. When they saw *my* determination, they jumped on board and helped me stay the course. In fact, some of them, like my cousin Bobby, have asked me to help them get started.

Another friend, Omar, who has known me and my brothers for years, was so impressed with my progress that he started working on himself—starting with cutting out fast foods. He's become one of my staunchest supporters . . . and he's following his own strict fitness program.

Ask your parents for their help. You may find out, as I did, that they've been wanting to help you lose weight but never knew quite how to approach you about the subject. I guarantee you they've been worried about your health. Maybe they never said anything about it because they were afraid they might hurt your feelings and sink you into a deep depression that will have you reaching for the Krispy Kremes and gaining more weight.

It's very important that you ask your parents to set up an appointment with your doctor, so you can start your diet and work out with a clean bill of health. The

That's me in the middle—with my round face, chubby cheeks, and double chin— enjoying the surf and sand at Miami Beach. I was only six or seven, but my mom already knew I was carrying more than baby fat.

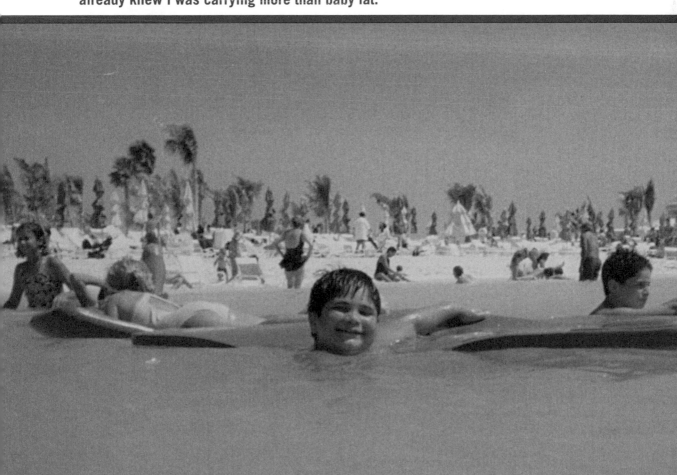

truth is, obesity may have caused damage to your body. Even kids as young as eleven or twelve are being diagnosed with type 2 diabetes, the kind that used to be known as adult-onset diabetes. That needs to be taken into account when you start a diet as well as when you begin an exercise program. Exercise changes how your body burns calories and can affect your blood-sugar levels. If your blood sugar level gets too low or too high, you can pass out, and it can lead to serious illness. Lugging around a lot of excess weight also damages your joints, another condition that must be monitored as you begin to exercise.

Your own doctor, like Dr. Rucker who has taken care of me and my brothers since we were small, may have some good ideas about how your mom and dad can support you as you lose weight. He or she may also be able to direct you to a nutritionist or even a diet plan that can be your guide as you restructure your diet.

After all, you are just one person in a whole family, and it's not very likely that the entire family will go on a diet just because you are. Even if there are others in your family who need to lose weight too, you may have to start out on your own.

If that's the case, you may need to step in and take control of your *own* meals. Either cook for yourself or ask your mom or dad, whoever's cooking your meals, to go easy on the spaghetti and meatballs, to stop bringing home the buckets of Kentucky Fried Chicken, and to drive right by McDonald's and Burger King. Ask if they can buy lettuce, tomatoes, carrots, and other things for you to put in a salad instead. You can stick to that while everyone else has mac and cheese.

When I first started, I was very, very rigid about what I ate and what I wouldn't, but, now that I've reached a size where I feel comfortable in my skin, I don't have to be so strict anymore. I've added a variety of foods—like the occasional bowl of pasta or a sandwich of whole grain bread—but I still keep tight control over the size of my portions. Second helpings are still a thing of the past.

The great thing is that, since I've learned completely new eating habits and have integrated exercise into my everyday life, I don't doubt that I'll be able to stay fit. The very idea of pigging out is not even a consideration.

IT'S BETTER THAN A GOOD IDEA

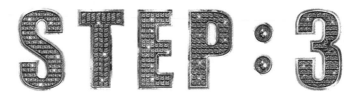

MAKE THE MIND-BODY CONNECTION

Once you've faced the fact that your weight is a problem and decided to get serious about losing it, and once you have lined up a network of support to hold you to your commitment, get ready to take your third step:

STEP 3: MAKE THE MIND-BODY CONNECTION

In short: Separate your self-worth from your body image.

That's not some silly slogan printed on a T-shirt, but it *is* an important piece of any successful weight loss puzzle.

You are not what other people say about you, but you are who *you* say you are. If you're not careful, you might start believing any insults hurled your way and start to identify yourself as "Fat Boy" or as the lard-ass loser that girl in school said you were when she refused to invite you to her party.

You may actually forget that you're simply a smart, funny, fun-loving, talented person who could stand to lose some weight.

Examine how what others say affects how you think of yourself. One of the most difficult lessons a person can learn: **What other people think of me is none of my business.**

Sure, I want people to like me—who doesn't?—and I want to fit in, but I don't want to be prejudged by my appearance or my size before people get a chance to know me. I want to be thought of as someone who is intelligent, a strong athlete, a kind person, a good man. What I'm trying to say is that my weight, no matter what it is, does not define me as a person, and anyone who thinks that it does is probably not someone I'll want to be around for long.

The important thing is that, in the course of losing weight, I have learned that *I* don't feel good—or feel good about myself—when my weight is out of control. I don't move as fast or as well as I do when I'm fit. I don't have as much energy either.

I have also learned that the more attention I pay to how my body *works* and how it feels physically—not just how it looks—the more I am able to focus my energy on its overall condition.

When it's getting close to mealtime, when I am deciding what I want to eat, I know almost instinctively what my body is asking for.

If I'm running low on energy, I may eat some fruit as a snack. Fruit offers a boost of natural sugar that raises my energy level and keeps it there, unlike candy and ice cream which give me that "sugar rush" that doesn't last very long and then drops out from under me.

If I'm tired, like all I want to do is go to sleep, my body seems to tell me it wants protein, like a piece of steak and leafy green vegetables that are high in iron and other nutrients.

And I know my mom's glad that every time she looks into the kitchen I'm not standing in front of the open refrigerator door, staring blankly into the space or nibbling on a bit of this and a little of that, in hopes of finding something that might tease my taste buds or stop the gnawing in my gut.

This is not woo-woo voodoo. It's simply a mind-body connection, just like the connection I make when I'm exercising and find myself slowing down halfway through my work-out. When that happens, I concentrate and focus my energy on the muscle group or groups I am working. By plugging into my body this way, I become re-energized and revitalized. The power of the mind over the body is amazing.

THERE'S NOTHING MAGIC ABOUT WEIGHT LOSS

I don't have any magical talents and I certainly don't have super powers that enabled me to zap the weight off. I don't need them and neither do you.

Losing weight is not all that different from making up your mind that you're going to go out for varsity football. You may not know if you'll be able to make the team, but you've decided it's possible for you to do it. You'll discover *how* to do it along the way. You train, and you start to eat right. You work out. Practice, practice, practice . . . then, eventually, you learn the ins-and-outs of the game and perfect your skills. You concentrate your energy, and, ultimately, you're ready to try out for the squad. Maybe you make the first team; maybe, junior varsity . . . but either way, you're in the game. And, as long as you're playing, there's a chance you'll win! The first step is to get out there on the field.

The most important thing you can do for yourself is to know that weight loss is possible, and then stay really, really flexible about where the process will take you. According to Jayne Tear, a New York-based consultant and educator who specializes in body management issues, you need to get away from the idea that you have to know *how* to lose weight before you do it.

Ms. Tear, who coaches people of all ages on how to gain control over their bodies, especially where obesity is concerned, says to tell yourself that you know that you are going to lose the weight. Just say, "I don't know how, but I'm going to do it."

You can trip yourself up if you're already thinking about *how* you are going to accomplish something before you have completely made up your mind that you are going to do it. This applies to anything, by the way, be it acing an exam or losing a certain amount of weight in a specific amount of time. Ms. Tear explains, "When you have *no doubt* that you are going to achieve something—such as losing weight— the process, or how you're going to do it, becomes an interesting discovery. You don't have to know how you're going to lose weight, only that you are. The 'how' of the matter will become clear along the way."

In short, you don't have to know *how* to lose weight, you simply need to determine *that you are going to do it.*

In all of the workshops and counseling she has done for people who have issues with their weight, never once has Ms. Tear recommended a specific diet or exercise plan to anyone. She sees weight loss, as a matter of "body management" rather than controlling your diet and exercise.

As Ms. Tear, who was a fat kid herself, explains it: "When I made up my mind to lose weight, I wasn't using willpower or self-motivation. I really *knew* it was possible for me to lose the weight, even though when I started I wasn't sure of how I was going to do it."

I know exactly what she means.

Once I made up my mind to lose weight, that's when I started to connect with my body and discover what I needed to eat to lose weight and stay healthy. I also began to experiment with exercises that would help me get cut and fit. Never once did I give up the notion that, by the time shooting started for the first season of *Growing Up Gotti*, I would be in shape . . . or almost there. And I was.

WATCH OUT FOR THE DOUBT TRAP

If you take something on, be it losing weight or going out for a varsity team, without a sense of absolute certainty that you will reach your targeted outcome, you can be sure that doubts will come up. Then you really will lose sight of your goal. You will get hung up on what diet you're going to try this week or the kind of exercise are you going to do next. You'll ask yourself if you really are good enough to make the squad or if you'll just end up sitting on the bench all season.

It's as if the conversations you're having in your head have taken over, and you've become so busy trying to determine the *how* of some task or so focused on the road head, you have lost sight of your target.

When you have no doubt about the outcome, any changes or uncertainty about the *process* will not alter this *outcome*. Keep your eye on the prize. Whatever glitches you encounter along the way will have no affect on your ultimate outcome.

As I did, you *will* lose weight.

However, if you have the preconception that the outcome has to be done a certain way, in a specific manner—like there's only one kind of diet or one type of exercise that will enable you to get fit—you will fail as soon as that process hits a snag. You will start to doubt your ability to produce your results, and you'll quit before your body has time to reap the benefits of your vision.

If you have a history of failed results—diets you've blown, exercises programs that failed—remind yourself that that was then, and this is now. Your past has nothing to do with your decision to lose weight *now*.

Keep telling yourself that your past has nothing to do with your future. Quit talking to yourself about the things that have failed you before. When you are managing your body, you are only moving forward.

Now, you're ready to go on to Step 4: Examine Your Eating Habits.

CIAO CHOW

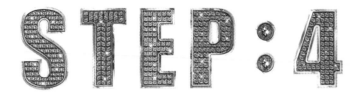

EXAMINE YOUR EATING HABITS:

THE WHAT, WHEN, WHERE, AND WHY

Let's get serious: If you weigh more than is healthy for your age and body type, then you are eating more than your body needs to sustain itself at that desired weight.

That being the case, it makes sense that if you eat only the amount of food your body needs to *maintain* your target weight, you will begin to lose the extra pounds and ultimately you will reach your goal, whatever it may be.

What could be more logical? The concept is so obvious it's embarrassing that this formula wasn't common knowledge to me.

So what is your ideal weight? You can look at the height and weight charts in your doctor's office, but that doesn't always take into account your age and body type. The school nurse or your coach, if you're on a team, may have one too, possibly one geared to adolescent boys and girls. You can even ask someone who is about your age and height and has the same body type as you—same shoulder and chest width but a smaller waist for example—and ask him what he weighs. Obviously, you weigh more than he does, so this will give you a weight for you to shoot for.

And rather than saying that is your ideal weight, let's say that it's your *target weight*, your desired ultimate outcome. Your own body will let you know when you've reached its *ideal weight*.

I knew that I was at least sixty, maybe seventy, pounds overweight when I started out. However, when I thought of losing that much weight all at once, it seemed impossible. It's not like I could strip off a sixty-pound fat suit, put on skinny clothes, and, in an instant, weigh what I wanted. So I figured I'd better give myself some intermediate weight goals—milestones—to make my weight loss more real and reachable.

I recommend picking a milestone you can visualize—say five pounds. Five pounds is a good milestone, especially early on in your diet experience, because you'll be able to feel a slight difference in the fit of your clothes. You can lose five pounds, and then another five pounds, and then another, and another until you've hit your target.

Just take care that you don't lose the *same* five pounds over and over again!

If you can't imagine what five pounds of flesh looks like, get yourself a visual aid. Go to the grocery store and check out the meat counter. Take a look at a five pound package of hamburger meat, a five pound roast beef, or a five pound ham.

When you've lost your first twenty pounds, reassess your weight loss goals. You may want to up that milestone to ten pounds!

Now let's talk about how you're going to lose these excess pounds. If you haven't studied it already in science class, a calorie is a measurement of energy. If you burn a tiny piece of coal, the amount of heat it releases is measured in calories. Our bodies work the same way, burning a specific quantity of food to release a certain number of calories.

Now, I'm not a nutritionist or scientist, so I won't go into a lot of explanation of calories consumed versus calories burned. So I've turned to the American Medical Association (AMA) for some guidelines. According to the AMA, a calorie (with a small "c") is a relatively tiny measurement. A Calorie—the capital "c" kind—is equal to 1,000 of the small "c" calories. It's the Calorie calories we're talking about when we're talking about the food we use to fuel our bodies.

It's enough to say that, if we are fat, we are routinely consuming more calories than our bodies can burn in a specific amount of time.

The number of calories you need depends entirely on how physically active you are. Generally speaking, because our bodies are not completely mature and because we are relatively active, we teenagers need a balanced diet of approximately 2,500 calories per day.

So what's a balanced diet? It's composed of a variety of foods from the three basic dietary components: protein, carbohydrates, and fats with protein and carbohydrate rich food packing more nutrition than fats. A balanced diet also "provides the body with all the vitamins and minerals it needs to thrive." For example, fresh green leafy vegetables, lima beans, and kidney beans provide folic acid, which helps produce red blood cells. Vegetable oils, wheat germ, whole grains, and dark green vegetables provide Vitamin E, which protect cells from damage and degeneration. The mineral chromium comes from meat, cheese, whole grain breads, and cereals to help the body burn carbohydrates. Iron, from meat, liver, eggs, and whole grain or enriched breads and cereals, delivers oxygen to the body tissues and is essential to the production of hemoglobin, the major component of red blood cells.

When you eat a variety of foods from a variety of sources—and I'm not talking about breakfast at Mickey D's, lunch with Wendy, and dinner with Arby either—you won't need to take vitamin and mineral supplements to stay healthy, not even a multi-vitamin.

Since your body can't distinguish if a calorie is from proteins, fats, or carbohydrates, you would be smart to choose foods that pack more punch than the empty calories of something like a bowl of ice cream or a jumbo order of fries. Even if you eat only good, nutritious foods it will be will be stored as fat if you consume more calories than your body needs to maintain your target weight.

Speaking for myself, when I decided to lose weight, I didn't weigh 179 pounds; I weighed 255. Obviously, I was eating enough to support my weight at 255 pounds instead of 179, so I had to cut back on how much I ate. That was the first component of the process I discovered to manage my body weight.

AIM FOR YOUR TARGET WEIGHT

So now you have a target weight—say it's 179 like my initial target—and you know that you need to consume about 2,500 calories per day while doing regular moderate exercise to reach that weight. Now it's time to get to work.

A word of warning: Don't become a slave to these numbers. Just let them be guidelines. Once you become familiar with appropriate portion sizes for specific foods and start to learn what foods provide you with the most nutrients for health, well-being, and weight loss, you will begin to know intuitively when you get close to that caloric ceiling for the day.

From my point of view, it wasn't just what I ate that got me fat, it was also how much I ate. And, because, to some extent, adolescents need more calories than adults. The difference is we need more carbohydrates, not more protein, to promote this growth.

Using the ballpark calories as a target, start reading labels and learning the calories *per serving size* in the foods you enjoy. Then plan a menu of these foods.

A word of caution: The serving size used to calculate the calories-per-serving of some foods can vary widely from what you or I might eat. Did you know that

Food—and lots of it—has always played a big part in my family's celebrations. Just look at the massive tray of cookies on the table at my birthday party when I turned nine or ten.

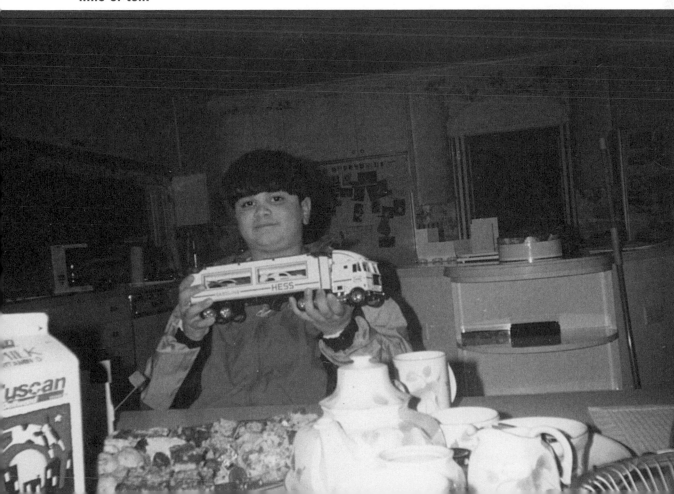

there are two and half servings in a twelve-ounce bottle of soda? Do you know of anyone who drinks just half a bottle of soda? I don't.

If you don't know where to look for the number of servings in a bottle of soda or on a box of cereal, check out the label. On the side or back of the package, you will see a box of numerals under the heading "Nutrition Facts." In it, you will find the calorie count, a breakdown of cholesterol, sodium, sugars, protein, and the various kinds of fat—saturated, polyunsaturated, and monounsaturated—and the ingredients, listed from the most to least. Toward the top of the box, after the name of the product, you will see two important lines: "Serving Size" and "Calories per Serving."

You may be in for a surprise. Did you know that two pieces of bread is not a serving?

A half-cup of plain old vanilla ice cream has about 170 calories. I don't know about you, I never ate just a *half cup*. For me, a serving size was more like the whole pint—and rarely did I have just vanilla.

Once you accept that one-level tablespoon of oil or shortening—a healthy extra virgin olive oil—butter, margarine, and even mayonnaise, has 120 calories in it, you will be less likely to float your salad in an ocean of vinaigrette. That's one *tablespoon*—not one cup!

A *three-ounce* grilled lean hamburger—no bun, no pickle, lettuce, tomatoes, cheese, or special sauce—has about 270 calories all by itself. That's an ounce short of a Quarter Pounder without cheese and all the other stuff that makes it taste so good. (The approximate calorie count for a Quarter Pounder with cheese is five hundred.)

Just three ounces of steak has about 254 calories and two all-beef hot dogs have roughly 320—without the buns and fries.

NO JOKE ABOUT CALORIES

The joke is that your body can't distinguish whether the calories come from a massive salad with tomatoes, carrots, celery, and mozzarella topped with slices of grilled chicken breast and three tablespoons of a light olive oil vinaigrette or chocolate-chocolate ripple ice cream with chocolate sauce and nuts. It's up to you to choose foods that nourish your body to the max.

And, because a calorie is a calorie, *all* excess calories—regardless if they come from protein, carbohydrates, or fatty foods—will be converted to fat. (The calories are stored in the fat cells of your body if you consume more than your body burns during the course of a day. So it's up to you to eat only the number of calories needed to fuel your body and maintain its ideal body weight. And it's up to you to use the highest octane fuel you can get.

Since I'm not a doctor, nutritionist, or scientist, I'm not about to go into great detail about counting Calories, calories, fat grams, net carbs, or any other specific diet plans. But I can share with you is what has worked for me. After all, I am an expert on my own weight loss. I quit eating fried food, bread, pasta, potatoes, and desserts; I gave up second helpings and between meal snacks, and I drank a lot of water and ate a lot of salad.

If you know anything about dieting, you know that you can't stick to a plan that is based on depriving yourself of all the food you love. Nevertheless you realize that dieting is pretty common sense, middle-of-the-road stuff. The point is you don't need an extreme diet to take off the pounds.

However, you may find that you need a more structured way of eating. If that's the case, ask your mom or someone whose judgment you trust to help you find one that will work for you. You can even hit the Internet to do your home-work. Check out Weight Watchers, Atkins, the Zone, and the other recognized programs. Whatever plan you choose, make sure it includes food that you like—and you will eat—and that it suits your lifestyle. If it says you have to eat special food at certain times during the day, and you have a heavy class schedule, and your school doesn't allow students to eat in the halls between classes, that diet could be a problem.

When you plan your diet, you'll want to choose foods that have the lowest number of calories and the largest serving size. That makes sense, doesn't it? You don't want to feel hungry, but you don't want to pack on the pounds either. As you change your eating habits, you will learn what makes you *feel* full, what gives you the most energy . . . and what slows you down.

I learned early on that if I ate a large salad with a light dressing, my stomach felt full, but I didn't get that uncomfortable or stuffed feeling. I got an energy boost from protein foods—a small steak, a grilled chicken breast or veal cutlet, even a slice or two of cheese. I drank plenty of water, too. Not only does water give you a feeling that your stomach is full, it also hydrates your skin, and it flushes toxins from your system. That's important as you burn calories and lose weight.

Since the nutritional value of different foods is not equal on a per calorie ba-sis, it's up to you to decide on a balance that gives your body what it needs.

You won't find the calorie count on any of the recipes you'll see in Chapter 11: "Recipes For Successful Weight Loss." These are some of the dishes I eat and enjoy. And I can cook many of them myself.

I'm not even going to launch into a long-winded discussion of the concept of "ideal weight." I'll leave that to a nutritionist or your family doctor—the experts. It can be pretty subjective, based more on your own sense of your body than what any chart can tell you.

What I will discuss is what I have found to be an underlying cause of overeating among teenagers.

Most people—guys anyway—eat what's put in front of them and never give it a thought. They eat what they like and skip what they don't. And, if they're "normal," they stop eating when they're full.

I wasn't wired that way. I never knew how to stop eating when I felt full. Instead, I ate until I felt *stuffed*, not just full, and even then I often kept on eating. I was out of control. Like, why did I eat that? Because it was there. No other reason. It was like being a foodaholic!

I suppose food had become my emotional security blanket during a time of stress in my family, starting with my parents' divorce, and, a few years later, the death of my grandfather and his very public funeral. At least there were no TV cameras following me around then like they are now. I would have been seen stuffing my face in almost every frame.

STEP 4: EXAMINE YOUR EATING HABITS: THE WHAT, WHEN, WHERE, AND WHY

By "examine" I mean that you should take a close look into when and where you eat, what you're eating and how much, as well as *why* you are eating. For example, if you're on the way home from school at three o'clock on Monday (that's the when), and you stop by the pizza shop (that's where), and you eat three pieces of sausage pizza with extra cheese (that's what you ate and how much), then it's time to look at the why.

Could it be that the only reason you ate pizza at three o'clock in the afternoon is because you and your friends *always* stop for pizza on your way home from school? Are you really hungry, or are you simply unconscious of why you eat then? Is it just something to do? Didn't you just have lunch during fourth period? That was barely two hours ago? Could your body possibly *need* three pieces of fatty sausage and molten cheese on yeasty dough to make it through until dinner time?

So, ask yourself, "How do I feel when I eat that much food so soon after lunch? Am I really hungry?"

I know we don't ordinarily get all tied up with our feelings, but in reality, this emotional component to obesity, and now weight loss, is critical.

I'm willing to bet that you will find that much of the nonmealtime food you consume is eaten unconsciously, maybe even in secret, out of the way of prying eyes. I also bet you're not really hungry either.

What are you thinking? That the food you eat when nobody's watching has no calories? Or that what you eat when nobody's looking or when you're standing at the counter at the pizzeria isn't real food . . . or that it doesn't count.

If you're a solo eater, maybe you're embarrassed for other people to see how much you're eating. The same goes for eating when you're out in a crowd. Could it be that you've convinced yourself that with seven or eight other guys hanging out and eating pizza, nobody will be paying attention to you—especially since you ordered your slices one at a time? Don't kid yourself. They know. Just look in the mirror, and you'll see what they see. They may not notice how much you eat while you're eating it, but there's no mistaking how much you've eaten when it shows up on your gut.

To a certain extent, it doesn't matter what the underlying cause is behind your secret eating; the only person you're fooling is yourself.

My goal is to help you discover what, when, and why you overeat to then help you learn what works for you to control your eating habits and to help you change your diet so that you *can* lose weight.

As you examine your food intake and your eating habits, consider your self-image. What do you think when you look at yourself in the mirror or when you see yourself in your school pictures? Slob, a loser, what?

Intellectually, all of us know that a person's weight is not a measure of his value as a person. Look at me! I didn't suddenly become a better person just because I lost more than seventy pounds. I was a good guy then, and I'm a good guy now. Too often we judge others unfairly by weight and size. Worst of all, we apply the same value judgements on ourselves too.

Being a teenager is hard enough without beating ourselves up about our weight.

GET A GRIP!

To get a handle on your own eating habits, I recommend that you keep a food diary for at least a week. Remember, you may see a pattern here. Exactly what do you eat? How much? Is it a twelve-ounce or sixteen-ounce steak, or a three- or four-ounce burger, without cheese, mayo, and bun? Do you eat seconds—and thirds—at every meal? Exactly how big are the servings of everything you eat? A mountain of mashed potatoes in a lake of gravy or just a hill and a puddle? Measure everything if you must, but don't lie.

Do you skip the green vegetables and salads for the fries and macaroni and cheese? Is there any fresh fruit in any given week? Do you drink milk, or do you drink cola at every meal?

Here's a sample of what a day's journal might look like. Go into as much detail as you can; just tell the truth. Especially about what—and how much—you eat and how you feel.

DAILY FOOD JOURNAL

DATE Friday, December 10, 2003

WHEN AND WHERE I ATE	WHAT I ATE . . . AND HOW MUCH	WHAT I WAS FEELING OR DOING
7:30 A.M. Home/car	Two chocolate iced doughnuts, can of cola	Breakfast—all I had time for
11:45 A.M. School	Two big slices of roast beef; mashed potatoes and extra gravy; three white rolls with butter; two cups of chocolate pudding; two containers of chocolate milk	Lunch This is what the lunchroom served that day.
3:00 P.M. Home Kitchen	Half leftover Chicken Parmesan hero; two Cokes	Snack I was hungry after school. Nothing else to do
5:00 P.M. Home My room	Three-quarters of a pint Ben & Jerry's Rocky Road ice cream	That's all there was in the freezer. Bored
6:00 P.M. Home Kitchen	Large bowl of penne with sausage and onions in tomato sauce; one fried, breaded chicken cutlet with mozzarella; 2 pieces of corn on the cob with butter; sautéed broccoli rabe with olive oil and garlic; three large glasses of Coke.	Dinner This is what Mom cooked for us.
8:30 P.M. My room	Ice cream sandwich (Vanilla ice cream with chocolate chip cookies)	Snack Bored—nothing on TV I wanted something sweet.
9:45 P.M. My room	Pint of chocolate chocolate-chip ice cream	Mom brought ice cream home. I was nervous about parents' divorce.

I can't begin to calculate how many calories I consumed in any one day! Looking back, all I can say is that's *a lot* of food!

Now get to work on your own Daily Food Journal.

DAILY FOOD JOURNAL

DATE_____

WHEN AND WHERE I ATE	WHAT I ATE . . . AND HOW MUCH	WHAT I WAS FEELING OR DOING

With every day you record your food intake, practice writing more and more details. How large was that hamburger? How much mayonnaise did you put on that bun? Cheese or not? How big was that serving of mashed potatoes, and how much gravy did you consume? Get specific, and tell the truth. These patterns can give you a sense of where you're making not-so-good food choices.

After seven to ten days—once you have recorded enough data to examine—go over your journal and highlight any patterns you see.

You may find that you eat a lot of potatoes—mashed potatoes with gravy at school; fries after school; and baked potatoes with butter, sour cream, and crumbled bacon for dinner a couple of nights a week—and notice that you have spaghetti one day, lasagna another, and rice and beans at school for lunch. The common denominator is starch—carbohydrates.

Carbohydrates—carbs—have gotten a lot of attention recently. Some people have even tried to eliminate them completely from their diets. You may hear these people saying they never eat "white foods"—no white bread, potatoes, pasta, rice, etc. The problem is that we need *some* carbohydrates for our bodies to generate vigorous energy.

The truth is our bodies need some carbohydrates to function at its best—just not as much as you probably consume. Carbohydrate foods provide the body with the fuel it needs for energy, and energy is what the body needs to burn calories. We simply don't need a diet that's *all* carbs.

In fact, breads, grains, rice, and pasta—all those tasty carbohydrates—stand at the base of the U.S. Department of Agriculture's Food Guide Pyramid, which examines the five major food groups—grains, vegetables, fruits, meats, milk produces and fats, oils, and sugars—and recommends the number of servings from each group your body needs per day to stay healthy. The original United States Food and Drug Administration (USFDA) Food Pyramid was introduced in 1992, and a new and improved version that supposedly considers all the new info unearthed in the past ten years is to be unveiled in 2005.

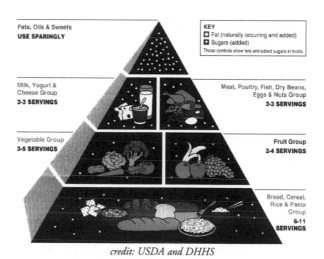

credit: USDA and DHHS

The pyramid form demonstrates how a variety of foods from each group is essential to a healthy, balanced diet, and when the initial pyramid was introduced, emphasis was on combating heart disease by stating that if you eat less fat, you will lower your cholesterol levels and have a healthier heart. The fat phobia that followed seemed to have no impact on heart disease and may have contributed to our national obesity problem. (We need some fats to encourage our bodies to burn the calories from carbohydrates and protein.) As if that weren't enough, it apparently kept people away from the good polyunsaturated and monounsaturated fats we need for health.

Research now shows that we don't need a large amount of fats, or even protein foods, either, but we need to be conscious of the calories in the food we eat. I'm not saying we need to obsess over calories, carbs, fats, or cholesterol, we just need to be aware of these values, so we can structure our food plans around the foods that give us the best nutritional boost.

The original USFDA Food Pyramid recommended between six and thirteen servings per day! To accomplish this you would have (1) a bowl of oatmeal or corn flakes with milk for breakfast, (2) a cup of chili with black or red beans, (3) a piece of cornbread for lunch, (4) four crackers with cheese for an after-school snack, and, for supper, (5) a cup of beef and barley soup, a grilled chicken breast, half cup of cooked spaghetti with marinara sauce, and a green salad with vinaigrette. You might even add a slice of whole grain bread to your dinner meal, if you still feel hungry. That's a LOT of food by any measure!

As you move up the Food Pyramid, the amounts of different foods you need get smaller, but the number of servings seem rather high, especially since we're in the middle of an epidemic of obesity.

Imagine having to consume two to five servings of vegetables; two to four of fruits and juices; two to three each of milk and milk products; and lean meats plus a bit of fats, oils, and sugars every day. Even I know that's a lot of food!

What I have discovered as I have learned to eat to lose weight and get fit is that I need to eat a variety of foods from every group. I just control the size of the portions I eat, and I make certain that I never let myself get too hungry.

The 2005 Pyramid will emphasize weight control—not just heart disease—and stresses the importance of regular physical activity in tandem with a balanced diet to lose weight.

It will also recommend that we consume between 20 and 35 percent of our daily calories from fats, acknowledging the benefits of monounsaturated and polyunsaturated fat.

Rather than stressing consumption of "complex carbs," new recommendations discuss the benefits of whole grains while urging us to limit our sugar intake. The truth is, all carbohydrate foods become sugar as they are metabolized by the body.

Consider refined carbs, such as white bread and other refined starches—all of which behave as sugar in the body—as empty calories. They add calories without providing wholesome nutrients. (See what I mean when I say make better food choices?)

New research says we need much less protein than what was once thought. This includes protein from meat, poultry, fish, nuts, and beans—including soy products. Again, eat a variety of protein foods, so you'll get the benefits offered by each.

Unless you have a physical condition, such as diabetes, or special dietary needs, like lactose intolerance—you have trouble digesting milk or milk products—or an allergy to peanuts or some other food, eat a few servings from each food group to get the nutrients you need to be healthy and fit. If you're especially active or play sports, it's okay to up the ante and eat a little more from the major groups.

Bread, Cereal, Rice, and Pasta Group

This group anchors the Food Guide Pyramid, so the foods in this group should make up the largest part of what you eat all day. That's because bread, cereal, rice, and pasta are all great sources of carbohydrates, the nutrients that the body uses as its major energy source. If you want lots of power, be sure to hit the bottom of the pyramid!

The catch is that your body turns these carb-rich foods into sugar, so it can generate energy. If that energy isn't used—if you sit around and play video games instead of working out or running around playing sports—you'll find the calories from carbohydrates quickly build up as fat on your body.

Again, if you're wondering what one serving is, it's not as much as you might imagine: one slice of bread; half a cup of cooked rice or pasta; half a cup of cereal; one ounce of cold cereal, or half a bagel or English muffin. *Note:* That's one half of a bagel or muffin, not one or two. If you want to eat an entire jumbo bagel consider that as at least two of your bread servings for the day.

Remember: A muffin the size of a softball, or a bagel or English muffin the size of a saucer, is more than one serving.

To pack more power into the foods you eat from this group, go for whole grain breads, cereals, and brown rice. They are far more nutritious than white foods like ordinary soft and white sliced loaf bread, quick-cooking white rice, pasta, and even instant oatmeal and cream of wheat.

Vegetable Group

You'll want to include three to five vegetables in your daily diet. Veggies are loaded with vitamins and minerals like iron and calcium. Carrots are a good source of vitamin A; beets contain iron and a natural chlorine that is known to flush fat out of your body, and tomatoes (which are really citrus fruits) and cauliflower contain vitamin C. Cabbage and Brussels sprouts are rich in sulphur and iodine, while broccoli, spinach, and other leafy dark green vegetables like kale, romaine, turnip greens, and collards are rich in iron, calcium, and a whole alphabet of essential vitamins.

Vegetables also provide carbohydrates for the energy your body needs, as well as plenty of fiber, which is important because it helps your digestive system do its job. They also contain plenty of vitamins and trace minerals.

Vegetables don't have to be raw for your body to get the benefits of the fiber either. Cooked vegetables have fiber too. Just don't overcook them, or you'll be throwing away the vitamins stored in them when you pour off the broth.

One vegetable serving might be one cup of raw leafy vegetables (although most eating plans designed for weight loss say you can eat as much lettuce—salad— as you want), half of a cup of other raw vegetables or cooked vegetables, or three quarters of a cup of vegetable juice.

Fruit Group

Fruit is vital to a balanced food plan—especially one geared for weight loss. The USFDA recommends two to four servings of fruit per day to get maximum use of important nutrients that keep you feeling healthy and looking good. Vitamin C is a big player in this food group—it's in fruits like oranges, strawberries, watermelon, and much more. Orange and yellow fruits (and vegetables too) are packed with antioxidants which are supposed to protect the body from a variety of diseases.

Bananas are a gold mine in potassium, which helps stop muscle cramps. That's a good thing to know if you're prone to charley horses. Fruits also give you carbohydrates, the body's favorite kind of fuel. And don't forget fiber: fruit is full of it. That helps with digestion.

Examples of what counts as one serving are one medium-sized apple, banana, orange, or tangerine; a half cup of cooked or canned fruit (preferably with no added sugar); three-quarters of a cup of fruit juice (like orange, grapefruit, or cranberry juice). You're better off eating a whole piece of fruit than drinking juice. A glass of fresh OJ, for example, may include the juice—and the calories—from three or even four oranges.

The Dairy Group

This food group, which includes milk, yogurt, and cheese, is close to the top of the pyramid. Even though these foods are important for good health, you don't need to consume as many of them in one day as you do of foods closer to the base of the pyramid.

If you listen to the dairy council, you'll be eating three dairy foods per day. That's not too much—but if you're watching your weight, you'll want to reach for the low-fat, no-fat, and reduced fat versions of each.

Milk, yogurt, and cheese fulfill your body's daily demand for calcium, which is essential for strong bones and teeth. Dairy foods also provide protein to help you grow and build body strength. They also provide a quick energy boost.

A suggested serving size is one eight-ounce glass of milk, one ounce of cheese (a piece about the size of your thumb), or one six-ounce container of yogurt.

The Meat, Poultry, Fish, Dry Beans, Eggs, and Nuts Group

Foods in this group are vital to a healthy diet; however, like milk, yogurt, and cheese, you don't need to eat nearly as much of them as you do of foods that are positioned lower down on the Food Pyramid.

The common denominator of the foods in this group—meats, such as beef, pork, and lamb; poultry, like chicken, turkey, and duck; fish, dry beans, eggs, and nuts—is that all of them supply you with the superimportant nutrient protein. They also load you up with iron, potassium, and zinc, among other vital vitamins and minerals. And, if you think dry beans belong in the carbohydrate category, you're right. They are high in carbs, too.

While the Food Pyramid suggests that people eat only two to three servings from this group daily, you don't have to go whole hog. Examples of what counts as one serving in this group are two to four ounces of cooked lean meat, poultry, or fish—that's a little smaller than the size of a deck of cards or the size of the palm of your hand. One ounce of meat is also equal to one whole medium or large egg; half a cup of cooked, dry beans (like pinto, black, or navy beans); 1 tablespoon of peanut butter or other nut butter.

The Fats, Oils, and Sweets Group

Fats, oils, and sweets are perched on top of the pyramid, which means that your body needs very little of them to stay healthy and fit. Your body does need some fats and oils for some very important bodily functions—like the metabolism of foods. It's like high octane fuel.

You just need to concentrate on getting the "good" kind of fat and oil, like the Omega-3 fatty acids, which have been found to reduce levels of cholesterol and triglycerides in the blood system and reduce joint pain. Omega-3s come from cold-water fish like salmon, white fish, ocean mackerel, anchovies, and herring. Meats, like beef, pork, lamb, and poultry, don't have these beneficial properties, which is why you need to include fish as well as meat in your diet.

Another oil/fat trap is trans fats, also known as trans-fatty acids. That's a liquid unsaturated fat that has been turned into a solid form through a process called "hydrogenation." Trans fat helps keep food fresher and adds to its flavor: Food producers developed hydrogenation in hopes of finding a substitute for the use of saturated fats—the kind that's used for frying—but it backfired.

Now research finds that the trans fat resulting from hydrogenation is potentially more damaging and dangerous that its predecessor. Just like saturated fat, trans fat is known to raise cholesterol levels and, more importantly, increases the "bad" LDL cholesterol.

Foods that guarantee you're eating too much hydrogenated fat are stick margarine; vegetable shortening, like Crisco; animal-based shortening, like lard; crackers, doughnuts, and cookies; all kinds of chips, pastries, and other commercially manufactured baked goods; most store-bought salad dressings; tortilla and taco shells, and many other foods we all eat such as ordinary grocery-store brands of peanut butter and microwave popcorn. Sorry, that's how it goes.

If you can't live without the taste of butter or margarine, use the soft kind that comes in a tub or liquid margarine unless the label says "trans fat free."

I don't have to remind you to avoid fried foods and junk pastries forever. When cooking, use liquid vegetable oils, like olive, safflower, canola, or corn oils.

There's a debate in the butter versus margarine controversy. I can't say to avoid butter and use margarine or vice versa. Whichever you use, the calorie count is the same.

I'm all for compromise: use a healthy vegetable oil like corn, canola, or olive for cooking and finish the dish with a teaspoon or two of real butter just at the end of the cooking process. This way you'll have that rich, buttery taste, without the unwanted fat and calories.

Sugary foods like candy and cookies are simple carbohydrates that can give you quick energy. They are usually loaded with empty calories and offer little or nothing in the way of nutrients. Just don't eat them. When I started my diet, those were the first things I quit eating.

In the right amount, though, fats and sweets can enhance the taste of food. When it comes to losing weight, the right amounts, according to the Food Pyramid, are very small. Still, rather than making yourself crazy wondering if you're eating too much butter, fat, oils, or sugar, cut out anything fried; don't add butter to anything, which won't be too awful since you're not eating baked potatoes and bread anymore, and stay away from sweet snacks and desserts.

That's not really as bad as it seems at first. Since I've began to cut sweets from my own diet, I have actually lost my taste for sweet things like ice cream, colas, candy, and pastries. I just don't want them anymore. Not long after I started my diet, I found that I really needed some guilty pleasures—tasty treats—to keep me from feeling deprived. Now I find that I prefer things like watermelon—cut it into cubes, remove the seeds, stick it into the freezer—which makes a great frozen fruit bar. I'm also big on strawberries to please my sweet tooth. Occasionally, as a special treat, I'll have a scoop of fruit sorbet.

FIGURING OUT THE NUMBERS

To give you an idea of the calories in foods we commonly eat, this chart might be a help. In addition to calories, it also lists the number of carbohydrate grams, the total grams of fat, and the amount of cholesterol per serving. I compared the information from several reliable resources and picked "ballpark numbers," so, if you decide that strict calorie, carbs, and fat gram counting is the only way for you to lose weight, check out the Internet or the Diet and Nutrition section at your neighborhood book store.

CALORIES, CARBS, FATS, AND CHOLESTEROL IN MANY FOODS WE EAT

FOOD	CALORIES	CARBS	FAT	CHOLESTEROL
BREAD				
Bagel, plain, 3.7 oz.	280	56 g	1.5 g	0 mg
Bread, white, 1 slice	110	20 g	1.5 g	0 mg
French toast 1 piece	245	17 g	7 g	95 mg
Pancakes, 3 medium	210	50 g	3.5 g	20 mg
CANDY				
Candy corn, 1 oz.	110	27 g	0 g	0 mg
Caramel, 6 pieces, 1.3 oz	160	27 g	5 g	5 mg
Chocolate, 1.7 oz. package M&Ms	240	34 g	10 g	5 mg
Chocolate, 1.9 oz. Mounds	250	31 g	13 g	0 mg
Chocolate, 1.5 oz. Hersheys	230	25 g	13 g	10 mg
Chocolate, 1.2 oz. Reese's peanut butter cup	180	19 g	10 g	0 mg
CEREALS				
Cereal, 1 cup, dry Cornflakes	100	24 g	0 g	0 mg
Cereal, 1 cup, dry Crisp Rice	120	29 g	0 g	0 mg
Cereal, 1 cup, hot oatmeal	150	27 g	3 g	0 mg
DAIRY				
Cheese, 1 oz. American	100	0 g	9 g	25 mg
Cheese, 1 oz. cheddar	110	0 g	10 g	30 mg
Cheese, ½ cup, cottage	120	5 g	5 g	25 mg

FOOD	CALORIES	CARBS	FAT	CHOLESTEROL
Cheese, ½ cup, Mozzarella, shredded	80	1 g	6 g	10 mg
Cheese, 1 tbs. Parmesan	20	0 g	1.5 g	0 mg
Cheese, 1 oz., Swiss	100	1 g	8 g	25 mg
Cream, 1 tbs., half & half	20	1 g	1.7 g	8 mg
Cream, 2 tbs., sour	60	1 g	5 g	20 mg
Cream, 1 tbs., whipped	30	0 g	3 g	10 mg
Milk, 8 oz., whole	150	12 g	8 g	35 mg
Milk, 8 oz., 2 percent	130	13 g	5 g	20 mg
Milk, 8 oz., skim	90	14 g	0 g	4 mg
Milk 8 oz. whole, chocolate	235	28 g	9 g	40 mg

DESSERTS

FOOD	CALORIES	CARBS	FAT	CHOLESTEROL
Cheesecake, ⅛" cake, cherry	400	55 g	12 g	35 mg
Cheesecake, ⅛" cake, plain	520	44 g	35 g	140 mg
Cookies, chocolate chip, 3 1-oz.cookies	160	22 g	7 g	10 mg
Cookies, oatmeal-raisin, 1.4-oz.cookie	180	30 g	6 g	10 mg
Cookies, Oreos, 3 ½-oz. cookies	160	23 g	7 g	0 mg
Doughnut, 1 3-oz. chocolate	320	35 g	19 g	0 mg
Ice Cream, ½ cup, chocolate	270	22 g	18 g	115 mg
Ice Cream, ½ cup, vanilla	180	15 g	8 g	25 mg

FISH

FOOD	CALORIES	CARBS	FAT	CHOLESTEROL
Salmon, 4 oz., broiled	206	0 g	9.2 g	81 mg
Shrimp, 4 large, boiled	22	0 g	0.2 g	43 mg
Tuna, 3 oz. steak	175	0 g	1.5 g	68 mg
Tuna, ¼ cup, canned/drained	65	0 g	0.5 g	30 mg
Tuna Salad, ⅓ cup	175	9 g	12 g	20 mg

FOOD	CALORIES	CARBS	FAT	CHOLESTEROL
FRUITS				
Apple, medium	80	21 g	0 g	0 mg
Apple Juice, 8 oz.	120	29 g	0 g	0 mg
Applesauce, ½ cup	100	27 g	0 g	0 mg
Banana, 1 medium	110	27 g	0 g	0 mg
Grapefruit, ½ medium	60	16 g	0 g	0 mg
Orange, 1 medium	65	16 g	0 g	0 mg
Strawberries, 8 medium	45	12 g	0 g	0 mg
Watermelon, ½ cup, cubes	23	5.7 g	0.3 g	0 mg
MEAT & POULTRY				
Bacon, 2 slices	90	0 g	7 g	15 mg
Beef, 4 oz., chuck roast	412	0 g	29.2 g	112 mg
Beef, 4 oz., ground	328	0 g	23.5 g	102 mg
Beef, 4 oz., sirloin	307	0 g	19 g	102 mg
Bologna, 2 slices	160	2 g	15 g	45 mg
Chicken, 4 oz., roasted breast with skin	220	0 g	12 g	83 mg
Chicken, 3 oz., roasted thigh with skin	153	0 g	9.8 g	58 mg
Chicken, 4 oz., breast, fried	435	49 g	26 g	65 mg
Chicken, 3 oz., boneless, grilled	196	0 g	5.5 g	96 mg
Eggs, 1 cup hard boiled, chopped	210	1.5 g	14.5 g	578 mg
Eggs, 1 large, poached	74	0.6 g	5 g	212 mg
Frankfurter, 1 all-beef	160	3 g	16 g	35 mg
Ham, 2 oz., deli sliced	60	2 g	1 g	25 mg
Pork, 4 oz., loin chops	220	0 g	12 g	45 mg

FOOD	CALORIES	CARBS	FAT	CHOLESTEROL
Pork, 4 oz., shoulder roast	200	0 g	15 g	50 mg
Pork, 4 oz., tenderloin	110	0 g	4 g	55 mg
Sausage, 3 oz., 1 Italian link	290	0 g	25 g	65 mg
Turkey, 4 oz., white	174	0 g	3.7 g	78 mg
Turkey, 4 oz., dark	212	0 g	8.2 g	96 mg
Turkey, 4 oz., deli	120	0 g	1.5 g	40 mg
Veal, 4 oz., cutlet	210	0 g	9.5 g	128 mg
Veal, 4 oz., chop	256	0 g	7 g	141 mg

NUTS AND BEANS

FOOD	CALORIES	CARBS	FAT	CHOLESTEROL
Baked beans, vegetarian, ½ cup	150	27 g	1 g	0 mg
Peanut butter, 2 tbs.	195	6 g	16 g	0 mg

OILS AND BUTTER

FOOD	CALORIES	CARBS	FAT	CHOLESTEROL
Butter, 1 tbs., salted/unsalted	100	0 g	11 g	31 mg
Margarine, 1 tbs.	100	0 g	11 g	0 mg
Mayonnaise, 1 tbs.	100	0 g	11 g	5 mg
Salad dressing, 2 tbs., oil/balsamic	145	2 g	16 g	0 mg
Salad dressing, 2 tbs., Bleu cheese	175	2 g	17 g	20 mg
Salad dressing, 2 tbs., Caesar	145	1 g	15.5 g	5 mg
Salad dressing, 2 tbs., French	140	8 g	12 g	0 mg
Salad dressing, 2 tbs., Italian	150	1 g	16 g	0 mg
Salad dressing, 2 tbs., Ranch	150	2 g	14 g	0 mg

RICE AND PASTA

FOOD	CALORIES	CARBS	FAT	CHOLESTEROL
Macaroni and Cheese, 1 cup	275	41 g	8 g	20 mg
Pasta, 2 oz., dry, all types	200	42 g	1 g	0 mg
Pasta sauce, ½ cup, Alfredo	200	17 g	15 g	50 mg

FOOD	CALORIES	CARBS	FAT	CHOLESTEROL
Pasta sauce, ½ cup, marinara	100	9 g	6 g	0 mg
Pasta sauce, ½ cup, meat	125	17 g	2 g	10 mg
Pasta sauce, ½ cup, pesto	200	2 g	24 g	0 mg
Pasta sauce, ½ cup, tomato	90	9 g	5 g	0 mg
Pasta, 1 cup, primavera	225	38 g	12 g	15 mg
Rice, ¼ cup, dry, brown	170	37 g	0 g	0 mg
Rice, ¼ cup, dry, white	170	36 g	0 g	0 mg

SOUPS

FOOD	CALORIES	CARBS	FAT	CHOLESTEROL
Soup, 1 cup, chicken noodle	100	8 g	2.0 g	10 mg
Soup, 1 cup, chicken rice	100	10 g	2.9 g	5 mg
Soup, 1 cup, tomato	120	27 g	0 g	0 mg
Soup, 1 cup, veggie beef	120	16 g	5 g	5 mg

VEGETABLES

FOOD	CALORIES	CARBS	FAT	CHOLESTEROL
Asparagus, 5 spears, fresh	25	4 g	0 g	0 mg
Avocado, ½ cup cubes	120	18.1 g	11.5 g	0 mg
Broccoli, ½ cup florets	22	3 g	0.2 g	0 mg
Broccoli rabe, 1 cup	30	3.9 g	0 g	0 mg
Cabbage, ½ cup, shredded	9	1.9 g	0.1 g	0 mg
Cabbage, ½ cup, cole slaw	190	15 g	15 g	0 mg
Carrots, 7 raw (½ cup)	35	8 g	0 g	0 mg
Cauliflower, ½ cup, florets	30	6 g	0 g	0 mg
Celery, 2 stalks	20	2 g	0 g	0 mg
Corn, 5-oz., ear	123	20 g	1.7 g	0 mg
Cucumber, ½ cup, sliced	7	1.4 g	0.1 g	0 mg
Green beans, ½ cup, cooked	22	3 g	0.2 g	0 mg
Lettuce, 1 cup, iceberg	20	3 g	0 g	0 mg

FOOD	CALORIES	CARBS	FAT	CHOLESTEROL
Lettuce, 1 cup, mixed	20	4.9 g	0 g	0 mg
Lettuce, 1 ½ cups, leaf	15	4 g	0 g	0 mg
Lettuce, 1 cup, romaine	15	3 g	0 g	0 mg
Peas, ½ cup, green	60	24.9 g	0.7 g	0 mg
Peppers, ½ cup, green/red	30	7 g	0 g	0 mg
Potato, 1 medium, baked	120	51 g	0 g	0 mg
Potato, ½ cup, boiled	116	27 g	0.1 g	0 mg
Potato, ½ cup, mashed	111	17.5 g	4.4 g	10 mg
Potato, 1 cup, hash browns	75	16 g	0 g	0 mg
Potato, 1 cup, French fries	165	25 g	7 g	0 mg
Potato, 1 medium, sweet	118	27.6 g	0.1 g	0 mg
Potato, 1 oz., chips	155	15 g	10 g	0 mg
Spinach, 1½ cups, raw	30	10 g	0 g	0 mg
Spinach, ½ cup, cooked	27	3 g	0 g	0 mg
Tomato, 1 medium, sliced	29	5.7 g	0.4 g	0 mg
Zucchini, ½ cup, raw	9	1.8 g	0.1 g	0 mg
Zucchini, ½ cup, boiled	14	3.5 g	.05 g	0 mg

You may want to keep going with your food diary as you begin to eliminate the things you don't want to eat because they encourage weight gain. Again, this will help to keep you in touch with when and what you're eating,

When you start telling the truth to yourself, you'll realize you haven't been doing a very good job!

One look in the mirror says it all, as does how your clothes fit, especially when even your XXXL shirt isn't as roomy as it used to be.

You really can get a handle on when and how much you eat as you start your weight loss program. And, as you begin to eliminate foods from your daily diet, journaling will also be helpful to keep track of what you eat. Keep a log of *everything* that goes into your mouth. The more rigorous you are, the more you become *conscious*, not just aware, of how much you eat.

When I first started working on myself, my only goal was to lose weight. As I got into it, I realized I had to make some serious changes in when, what, and how I ate. I also had to find a balance in my diet, one that I could live with. I wanted to eat foods that I liked and made me feel good. As my mother often reminded me, I needed food that would provide my body with sufficient vitamins, minerals, and electrolytes so that I wouldn't find myself starving at the end of the day, and so that my body can grow stronger and healthier.

CRASH DIETING IS HAZARDOUS TO YOUR HEALTH

Do not, under any circumstance, crash diet! Fad diets and those over-the-counter weight-loss drugs sold in drug stores and blasted all over TV may promise quick weight loss, but they can be dangerously unhealthy. This is especially true for kids and teens.

Think of it this way. You didn't get fat overnight or even in a couple of months, so don't expect to lose your extra weight in a flash. Give your body time to adjust as you lose weight.

The truth is that, if you starve yourself by eating too few calories, you will cause yourself harm. Your body will think it's starving, and your metabolism will slow down, which makes further weight loss increasingly difficult. A body that's starving doesn't want to burn off all those calories that are stored in fat.

If you lose weight too quickly, this can also cause damage to your heart and other vital organs. You'll also find that your energy is zapped, and your ability to concentrate is zip. Your skin starts to look dull and dry, like you've never seen the sun, and your eyes will look lifeless. Your hair will become dull and flat, no matter what kind of shampoo and styling gel you use. The shine just won't be there. You are not healthy.

Quick weight loss followed by equally rapid weight gain is called yo-yo dieting and can screw up your body big-time. This pattern of starvation and rapid weight loss teaches your body that you're starving, so it quits burning calories with any efficiency. So, when you start overeating again or go back to eating less nutritious fatty foods, your body is reluctant to burn up the calories you're feeding it, so it all changes to fat.

Statistics say that most of us are overweight, with a large percentage being obese. A lot has been written about girls who have eating disorders, like anorexia and bulimia, or who are obese, but there is little written or said about guys who binge eat or starve themselves.

Boys may be different physically, but the damage caused by an unhealthy starvation diet is the same: listlessness, anemia, loss of focus and the inability to concentrate, irritability, headaches, hair loss, kidney stones, liver damage, and loss of muscle tissue and tone. Your skin will be dull and drab too, like you've been sick with the flu of something even more serious.

That's almost as frightening as the potential dangers inherent in being morbidly obese. Stay away from the extremes when it comes to your eating habits and dieting!

Ask for help from your parents, friends, anyone who will listen. Generate partnerships with your family members to support you in creating the best possible weight loss program for yourself. Ask the person who shops for groceries and cooks your family's meals to stock up on foods you can eat and leave the cookies, candies, and ice cream that will get you off track on the store shelves. You might even ask everyone to join you and experiment with eating healthy diet food. At the end of this book, I will give you some of the recipes I've eaten over the past year and a half. Believe me, they're easy enough for *anyone* to make.

Don't give up your diet before the miracle happens. I know how silly that sounds, but it's important to give yourself enough time to change your eating habits. If you don't, you'll surely go back to your old, unhealthy way of eating and regain every single pound you lost, if not more.

This is a great time to practice patience. Keep reminding yourself that you did not gain all that weight overnight, so you can't expect to lose it overnight either. And never, ever lose sight of your intended outcome.

MANGIA! MANGIA!

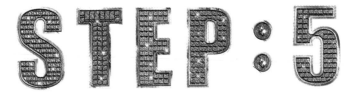

STEP : 5

LEARN TO MAKE BETTER FOOD CHOICES

By now you're on your way to learning the importance of eating to live rather than living to eat.

That's easy enough to do when you're eating at home where you can have some control over what goes into your meals and onto your plate, but you won't be able to eat every meal at home. What happens when you go out to eat with your family or when you're at school? And what happens when you go out on a date?

That's where the next step comes in, big time.

STEP 5: LEARN TO MAKE BETTER FOOD CHOICES

Now is the time to take what you've learned about eating and preparing food at home and apply this new knowledge and awareness to dining out. This includes eating at school.

Luckily, school lunch programs today offer healthy food choices. Find what you want to eat from there, and ignore the rest of the menu. As I mentioned, my own school has a salad bar. It's not particularly imaginative, but it's definitely a start.

I started eating in restaurants with my family when I was very young. I'm the chubby-cheeked six-year-old on the right—next to my dad. That's Carmine on the other side, in front of Bugs.

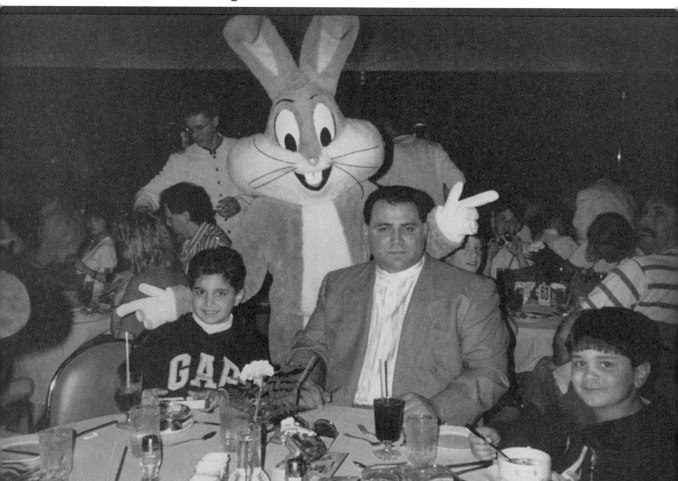

You'd have to have been living under a rock not to know that a steady diet of junk food isn't healthy, and it *will* make you fat, especially if you eat too much of it. Let's face it: If you eat too much of foods that are really good for you, you will gain weight too.

So, that said, it's up to you to learn what makes up a balanced diet. This could mean ordering a grilled chicken breast and green salad instead of the a double cheeseburger deluxe with a side of fried onion rings or joining the Colonel for the four-piece Original Recipe special with extra mashed potatoes and double gravy. It may be as simple as giving up bread, potatoes, and pasta.

HAVE A GAME PLAN BEFORE MEALTIME

You probably know, at least generally, what's on the menu, and you can probably figure out what's best for you to eat before you walk through the door of the restaurant or pull up to the drive-by. I can't say it enough: Have a game plan before you're so hungry, you lose your food objectivity.

These days, even Mickey D, Wendy, and the King are offering "diet" or "healthy" menu items. Look there first.

Just remember that these foods aren't always as low-cal as you might assume, but you really can eat them without fear, provided you use your head.

PLUSSES TO FAST-FOOD EATING

There's a plus side to eating in fast-food restaurants that I'll bet you never thought of. Because you order from the counter rather than sitting at a table with a basket of crackers and bread in front of you while the waiter races off to give your order to the kitchen, you won't be tempted by the nibbles before you start your meal.

- **Order foods with one of the following words in the title: "small," "junior," "medium," or "child's" in its name. (No, you will *not* be carded. The waiter won't care. There's no age limit on kids' meals.)**

- **Go for the grilled chicken rather than beef burger, fried chicken, or fish.**

- **Toss the top half, if not all, of the bun.**

- **Have it your way—*without* mayonnaise and special sauce.**

- **If you absolutely, positively *must* have fries, split a small order with a friend.**

- **Order a salad, no croutons or bacon bits, and ask for low-cal dressing on the side. (Then you can dip your salad into the dressing or just use half of what the waiter serves.)**

If you're like me, you like pizza, and, since you're dieting to lose weight, you're outright pissed that you can't eat it anymore. That isn't necessarily so.

In fact, pizza beats most burger-and-fries meals any day. While your average slice of cheese pizza is approximately 750 calories, that bacon double cheeseburger has 475 calories and the large fries 400. All you have to do is make some smart choices in ordering that slice. Here's how:

- Pizza can be made to order, so order it the way you want it.

- Order the thinnest crust on the menu. Run from any crust that's stuffed with cheese!

- Unless you're eating out with a crowd, don't buy the jumbo pie.

- Order a "plain" pizza—tomato sauce and cheese—without extra cheese. Extra cheese adds extra fat and calories you don't need.

- If you must have an extra topping, rather than getting pepperoni, sausage, or hamburger, choose a lean topping, like vegetables—mushrooms, garlic, onions, green pepper, olives, plum tomatoes—or sliced grilled chicken. Toppings add calories, fat, and sodium to your meal and jeopardize your new food plan. (A single slice of pepperoni pizza will have more than 1,000 calories—most of it from fat.)

- *Limit portion size.* Never eat more than two slices per meal, and never get a "personal pan pizza," or you'll be eating far too much for one meal.

- Supplement your pizza meal with a green salad topped with raw carrots, onions, cucumbers, and low fat dressing. You can make a full meal of one slice and a salad! I promise.

- Skip the bread sticks and garlic rolls.

- If there's any pie left over after you and your date have eaten your full, either ask the waiter to take it away or pack it into a doggie

**box and wrap it up. Get it out of sight, so you won't keep picking
at it.**

If you're eating at a sit-down restaurant where you've eaten before, decide what you're going to order before you walk in the door. That's not to difficult, since you are already familiar with the menu. Some restaurants even advertise specific diet menus—such as the Weight Watcher menu advertised by the Applebee's chain. This features recipes and portions that comply with the Weight Watchers program of counting points. Other restaurants and catering firms follow the food plans of some programs such as Atkins, South Beach, and The Zone diets, and many eateries designate foods that are "Heart Smart" in keeping with the guidelines set by the American Heart Association. You can count on these dishes to be low fat and, probably, low-cal.

If this is your first time in a place, don't worry. You *will* be able to eat without blowing your diet. If you're still dubious about being able to stick with your commitment to losing weight, call the restaurant in advance, and ask about their menu. You might even find the restaurant's Web page and see it for yourself.

- **Order an appetizer for your entrée. If you don't find something that fits with your food plan, ask for a half order or a child's plate of a dish you *can* eat.**

- **If a waiter gives you any grief, calmly explain that you have a food allergy. No one can argue with that. Besides it's true: you *are* allergic to high fat foods.**

■ Even if the menu says "no substitutions," don't hesitate to request the changes you need. Overeating is like any other food "allergy." It can make you feel sick.

■ Don't hesitate to ask for what you want and need to stay on your diet. Remember, you are the paying customer. It's to the restaurant's advantage to have you as a happy and satisfied customer, even if you're just a fourteen-year-old kid. What a smart way for a restaurant to cultivate a loyal, long-term customer.

■ You can also play the allergy card again if the waiter gives you grief about asking if a dish can be prepared the way you need it. No one can argue with an allergy. Besides it's true: You *are* allergic to high calorie foods.

■ Unless the people you're eating with object, ask that the bread sticks and rolls be taken off the table, so you won't be tempted to nibble. If not, keep your hands out of the basket. Bread sticks and rolls are nothing more than wasted calories.

■ Look for words like "grilled," "roasted," and "broiled" on the menu. Avoid anything that is "deep fried."

■ Avoid any dish described as "au gratin"—with cheese—or with creamy sauces. Otherwise, you're racking up unnecessary calories.

■ Ask if a sautéed or pan-fried dish can be cooked with little or no oil or if it can be grilled.

- Ask the waiter if the chef will *grill* or *broil* your meat entrée.

- If your meal comes with potatoes, ask for a side salad or a second vegetable like steamed broccoli and green beans instead. If you must have a potato, ask for a plain, baked potato—no butter, no sour cream, no bacon bits, and no gravy.

- Request that all sauces and salad dressing are served on the side. This gives you control of how much you eat.

- Steer clear of creamy salad dressings. If they don't have a plain vinaigrette, ask the server to bring olive oil and vinegar, so you can make your own.

If you go into an unfamiliar Italian restaurant, go lean and green. Ask if you can have that piece of veal or chicken can be broiled, with a brush of olive oil, no butter. Chicken Francese is sautéed and flavored with fresh lemon juice. Can it be sautéed without a lot of oil? What about having a Caesar salad with grilled pesto chicken or grilled salmon?

If you really can't bear the idea of depriving yourself of Spaghetti Bolognese, ask for a half order or child's plate, then fill up on salad.

Another way to make smart food choices while dining out is to familiarize yourself with the kinds of foods in the various cuisines. For example, if you're eating Chinese, stay away from the fried dumplings, egg rolls, and spring rolls. A cup of hot and sour soup is a filling and satisfactory starter. Avoid main dishes that include breaded or fried ingredients, such as General Tso's Chicken, which is fried pieces of chicken in a spicy sauce of onions, peppers, mushrooms, and chilies. Check out the chicken and steamed broccoli with garlic sauce. If you're not sure about an item on the menu, ask.

Going for Japanese? My favorite meal is a large salad and a California roll. Scratch teriyaki or any of the other fried entrees off your list.

When eating Mexican, order a taco salad with salsa instead of dressing, and don't eat the taco shell or taco chips. Order black beans or red beans; just make sure they're not refried.

Even your basic all-American diner can serve up a fitting diet meal. Sometimes they're listed under diet plates or something like that. Otherwise you can piece a great meal together on your own.

- Check out the salads. Cobb salad, Greek salad, chef's salad—ask what's in them. Then request that the dressing be served on the side. (Another tip: Dip your salad, one fork-full at a time, into the dressing rather than dousing your salad with it. You'll be able to enjoy the taste of the dressing and get fewer calories and fats.)

- Choose chopped steak (no gravy) with salad or cottage cheese over a burger deluxe platter or meatloaf with mashed potatoes and gravy. Ask them to hold the fried onion rings that are usually used as garnish unless you're sure you can resist the temptation.

- At breakfast time, ask for half a melon with yogurt or cottage cheese or a bowl of fresh fruit. (Make sure it's fresh; some restaurants put sugar-packed canned fruit cocktail into their fruit cups.) Another option is poached eggs on whole wheat toast and Canadian bacon—no butter and no potatoes. Remember, at most diners, you can order breakfast any time of day.

- When ordering steaks or chops, the key words to look for are grilled and broiled. Ask for double vegetables or a salad and vegetables— no potato—and hold the gravy, please.

- No matter what you have ordered, if the serving is especially large, ask for a take-out container *before* you start eating, wrap half of it to take home. Have it for lunch or supper the next day.

- Gotta have dessert? Make it a fruit bowl, without whipped cream or ice cream, or low-fat, low-cal frozen yogurt. If there's nothing "legal" on the menu—and you don't have the fortitude to pass up a sweet—order something and take *one* bite. Either give the rest away or ask that it be taken from the table.

If you stay cool, use your head, and order with your brain rather than with your eyes and urges, you will be able to stick to your weight loss program while eating away from home. With a little practice and concentration, it'll be almost as easy as when you're sitting at your own kitchen table.

The following chart is just a sample of some of the mainstays of some of the best-known fast food restaurants. If you don't find your favorite burger, pizza, or fried chicken listed, you can always go online and check out the chain's website for the full picture. If not, just go in and ask to see the nutritional breakdown of the menu. In some states, this information has to be posted in plain view, but if not, just ask.

I'm sure you'll be able to find plenty that you can eat wherever you go.

CALORIES, CARBS, FATS, AND CHOLESTEROL IN MANY OF THE FAST FOODS WE EAT

FOOD	CALORIES	CARBS	FAT	CHOLESTEROL
ARBY'S				
Big Montana Roast Beef	590	41 g	29 g	115 mg
Regular Roast Beef	320	34 g	13 g	45 mg
Grilled Chicken Deluxe	450	37 g	22 g	110 mg
Chicken Caesar Salad	230	8 g	8 g	80 mg
Large Fries	570	82 g	24 g	0 mg
BURGER KING				
Whopper with cheese	800	53 g	49 g	110 mg
Whopper Junior	390	31 g	22 g	45 mg
Double Whopper with cheese	1060	53 g	69 g	185 mg
Chicken Tenders, 5 pieces	210	13 g	12 g	30 mg
King Fries	600	76 g	30 g	0 mg
Chicken Caesar Salad	190	9 g	7 g	50 mg
Chocolate Shake, medium	600	97 g	18 g	70 mg
DAIRY QUEEN				
Grilled Chicken Sandwich	340	26 g	16 g	55 mg
DQ Homestyle Burger	290	29 g	12 g	45 mg
Chicken Strip Basket, 6-piece	1,120	102 g	60 g	60 mg
Medium Vanilla Cone	330	53 g	9 g	30 mg

FOOD	CALORIES	CARBS	FAT	CHOLESTEROL
DOMINO'S				
Ultimate Deep Dish 12" Cheese	238 per slice	28 g	11 g	11 mg
Classic Hand-Tossed 12" Cheese	186 per slice	28 g	5.5 g	9 mg
Crunchy Thin Crust 12" Cheese	137 per slice	14 g	7 g	10 mg
Ultimate Deep Dish 12" Pepperoni	275 per slice	28 g	14 g	19 mg
JACK-IN-THE-BOX				
Breakfast Jack	305	34 g	14 g	205 mg
Jumbo Jack with Cheese	695	55 g	41.5 g	70 mg
Chicken Fajita Pita	315	33 g	9 g	65 mg
Natural Cut Fries—large	530	69 g	25 g	0 mg
Chocolate Ice Cream Shake—small	660	89 g	29 g	110 mg
KFC (KENTUCKY FRIED CHICKEN)				
Original Recipe Breast	380	11 g	19 g	145 mg
Extra Crispy Thigh	370	12 g	26 g	120 mg
Chicken Pot Pie	770	70 g	40 g	115 mg
3 Colonel's Crispy Strips	400	17 g	24 g	75 mg
Mashed Potato with Gravy	130	18 g	4.5 g	0 mg
Coleslaw 5 oz.	190	22 g	11 g	5 mg
McDONALD'S				
Egg McMuffin	290	30 g	11 g	235 mg
Big Mac	560	46 g	30 g	80 mg
Filet-o-Fish	400	42 g	18 g	40 mg
Quarter Pounder	420	40 g	18 g	70 mg
6-piece Chicken McNuggets	250	15 g	15 g	35 mg

FOOD	CALORIES	CARBS	FAT	CHOLESTEROL
Large french fries	520	70 g	25 g	0 mg
Grilled Chicken Caesar	200	10 g	6 g	70 mg
McFlurry Oreo	560	88 g	16 g	50 mg
Triple Thick Shake—small chocolate	440	76 g	10 g	40 mg

PIZZA HUT

FOOD	CALORIES	CARBS	FAT	CHOLESTEROL
12" Sausage Lover's	330 per slice	29 g	17 g	30 mg
Hand Tossed Veggie Lover's	220 per slice	31 g	6 g	15 mg
6" Personal Pan Pizza with cheese	160 per slice	18 g	7 g	15 mg
12" Meat Lover's	340 per slice	29 g	19 g	35 mg
Stuffed Crust Meat Lover's	450 per slice	21 g	21 g	55 mg

SUBWAY

FOOD	CALORIES	CARBS	FAT	CHOLESTEROL
6" Classic Cold Cut combo	410	47 g	17 g	60 mg
6" Subway Club	320	47 g	6 g	35 mg
6" Cheese Steak	360	47 g	10 g	35 mg
Turkey-Breast Wrap	190	18 g	6 g	20 mg
6" Veggie Delite	230	44 g	3 g	0 mg

* Sandwiches made on Italian or wheat bread

TACO BELL

FOOD	CALORIES	CARBS	FAT	CHOLESTEROL
Chili Cheese Burrito	390	40 g	18 g	40 mg
Burrito Supreme Beef	440	52 g	18 g	40 mg
Gordita Supreme Chicken	290	28 g	12 g	45 mg
Regular Style Taco	170	13 g	27 g	55 mg
Grilled Steak Soft Taco	280	21 g	17 g	55 mg
Cheese Quesadilla	490	39 g	28 g	55 mg
Taco Salad, Fiesta, no shell	500	42 g	27 g	65 mg

FOOD	CALORIES	CARBS	FAT	CHOLESTEROL
Pintos 'n Cheese	180	20 g	7 g	15 mg
Enchirito Beef	380	35 g	18 g	45 mg
Nachos	320	33 g	19 g	4 mg

WENDY'S

FOOD	CALORIES	CARBS	FAT	CHOLESTEROL
Junior Hamburger	280	34 g	9 g	30 mg
Junior Cheeseburger	320	34 g	13 g	40 mg
Junior Cheeseburger Deluxe	360	37 g	16 g	45 mg
Classic Single, with everything	430	37 g	20 g	65 mg
Big Bacon Classic	580	46 g	29 g	95 mg
Grilled Chicken Sandwich	360	44 g	7 g	75 mg
Biggie French Fries	490	65 g	24 g	0 mg
Bacon-Cheese Potato	560	69 g	25 g	40 mg
Mandarin Chicken Salad	170	17 g	2 g	60 mg
Medium Frosty, 8 oz.	430	74 g	11 g	45 mg

WHITE CASTLE

FOOD	CALORIES	CARBS	FAT	CHOLESTEROL
Cheeseburger (1 sandwich)	160	11.0 g	9 g	15 mg
Hamburger (1 sandwich)	140	11.0 g	7 g	10 mg
Double Cheeseburger	290	16.0 g	18 g	30 mg
Bacon Cheeseburger	200	12 g	13 g	25 mg
Chicken Rings, 6 pieces	210	10.0 g	14 g	50 mg
Small Fries	115	15 g	6 g	0 mg
Onion Rings, 8 pieces	290	38.0 g	13 g	1 mg
Chocolate Shake	250	37.0 g	8 g	30 mg

GET MOVING!

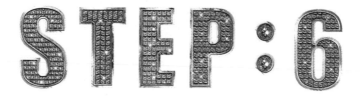

STEP : 6

GET TO THE HEART OF WEIGHT LOSS

WITH EXERCISE

There's a reason everyone talks about the importance of a diet and *exercise* program for healthy weight loss—especially for teens. Dieting alone does little to produce permanent weight loss. And permanent weight loss is exactly what I wanted for myself. I don't intend to ever, ever pack on the pounds again.

So this brings me to Step 6 of my program.

STEP 6: GET TO THE HEART OF YOUR WEIGHT LOSS WITH EXERCISE.

Believe it or not, exercise actually makes it easier to stick to a reducing diet. It is the "heart" that keeps your body pumping and burning calories on your way to health.

Take it from me, it's a myth that exercise increases your appetite. In reality, it's quite the opposite. The truth is that aerobic exercise, the kind that increases your heart and breathing rates, actually speeds up metabolism—that's what governs how efficiently your body burns calories—from four to eight hours after you've stopped working out.

This means that, if you've been doing active, aerobic exercise, like playing tennis, jogging, swimming laps, etc., your body will keep burning calories long after you've stopped.

Nonaerobic or anaerobic exercise, such as lifting weights, which I do regularly to build muscle mass, does not increase your metabolic rate to such a degree. It does, however, make your body leaner and stronger and helps to increase your stamina.

That's why I can say without a doubt that a balanced exercise program for effective weight loss requires both aerobic and anaerobic exercise.

Regular aerobic exercise has amazing benefits to the body. Exercise combats such physical problems as high cholesterol and high blood pressure, increases energy, eases stress, and that's just for starters.

Ideally, you need to do a combination of aerobic exercise and strength training to gain maximum fitness. The official definition of aerobic exercise, according to the American College of Sports Medicine (ACSM), is "any activity that uses large muscle groups, can be maintained continuously, and is rhythmic in nature." Basically, it's any exercise that causes the heart and lungs to work harder than they do when you are at rest, forcing them to work from sixty to eighty-five percent of their capacity.

You don't even need to do an aerobic workout every day. Experts contend that all you need for affective weight loss is to work out three times a week for between twenty and thirty minutes per day.

That said, phys-ed class two to three days a week is *not* enough exercise for a teenager to get fit and lose weight. We need a more active regimen. My doctor, Dr.

Playing lacrosse was a helpful way for me to burn up calories and create muscle tone. Here, I'm with my teammates. From left, Brian Yampol, Christian Walton, and Thomas Laviano, on our way to practice. Before I started losing weight, I was a good player; now that I'm no longer lugging around all that extra poundage, I'm a faster player as well.

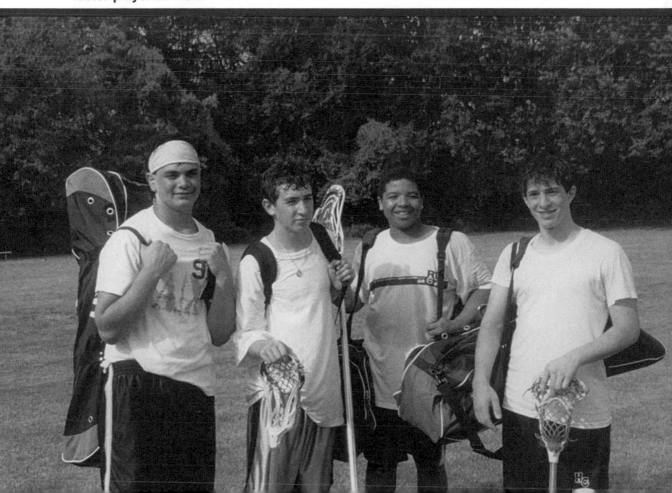

Rucker, whose medical practice treats children and adolescents, says that a regular after-school exercise program is essential to getting and staying fit, never mind how integral it is to losing weight.

You don't have to go out for varsity sports or even start kick-boxing or take a step aerobics class either. Moderately active exercises such as taking a thirty-minute walk every day or riding your bike to and from school two or three times a week can be quite effective.

Sometimes when I wake up in the morning, I'll ride my bike to and from a gas station a few miles away from my Long Island home. Our house is in the town of Old Westbury, and the gas station is nearby. It's a safe ride too. There's not too much traffic on these country roads. The round-trip ride not only burns calories, but it also builds up the muscles in my legs. It's a great way to start the day.

Early morning is the perfect time to exercise because it sets you up to start your day fully energized. If you have your workout too close to bedtime, it can give you so much energy that you'll have a hard time sleeping. That just goes to prove that exercise does *not* tire you out. Instead, it revs up your energy.

The most important component of aerobic exercise is that you find something you enjoy doing—and then do it regularly. Whatever you do, it should be a type of activity that keeps your heart rate elevated for a continuous period of time, and start moving.

And, whatever exercise you do, it has to be fun! If it's not, you won't do it for very long.

To find out if you're overdoing your aerobic exercise, take the "talk test." That is to say, if you are too out of breath to carry on a conversation while you're jogging or dribbling a basketball down the court, you are probably working too hard and need to pull back. Slow down, but don't come to a halt.

Of course, for maximum benefit from your exercise, you should be working hard enough to break a sweat, so don't cut back too much.

Other warning signs are chest pain—or any kind of pain for that matter—and dizziness. If that happens, slow down and slowly come to a stop. **Pain does not mean gain.** Pain is your body's way of signaling you that something is badly wrong. It's up to you to find out what has happened, so tell your parents, your teacher, or your coach.

If you think you want to run in the New York Marathon, start out slow—especially if you're in your early teens. Extreme distance running, like a marathon or triathlon, should *not* be attempted until you're absolutely sure that you are completely grown, and your bones and muscles are mature. As a rule, marathon organizers don't allow anyone under eighteen to enter. Until then, shoot for running a 5k race.

Moderate aerobic exercise—such as walking at about two miles per hour—about as fast as you rush between classes—burns approximately 198 calories per hour. Riding a bike at about five miles per hour burns roughly 175; if you speed up thirteen miles per hour, you'll be burning more than 610 calories an hour, and a game of touch football burns just under five hundred calories per hour.

Since you have to burn 3,500 calories to lose one pound, and since the average teen needs to consume a minimum of two thousand calories per day to stay healthy and lose weight, it stands to reason that to achieve any effective weight loss, you'd better get up and start moving. Lying around in front of the TV burns only eighty-five calories per hour, maybe less. And no, watching *more* TV doesn't make it healthier for you. FYI, adults over twenty-five years old should never eat *less* than one thousand calories per day. People, like us, who're under twenty-five, need that extra thousand calories to maintain our energy level, brain power, and overall health.

You see, there's another vital benefit to regular exercise. Unless you exercise while you diet, you can lose weight—and look slimmer—and still be too fat. This is especially true if you've lost the weight too quickly.

What happens is that, unless you're working out on a regular basis as you diet, you may have been losing muscle tissue instead of body fat.

In case you're curious about how fat your body really is, pinch a fold of skin from three places on your body:

- **The upper side of your upper arm.**

- **One side of your abdomen, near your hip bone.**

- **In the middle of the back of your thighs.**

Measure the skin you pinch. You can use a ruler if you don't have a caliper handy to do the job. Hey, not everyone's studying engineering, but your phys ed teacher or a trainer at the gym may have one. Body Mass Index (BMI)—the ratio of lean muscle to fat—is one of those things fitness experts are talking about these days.

If you can pinch an inch or less of flesh—in all three places—your body fat level is low to moderate. That is, it's okay. If you're pinching more than an inch, figure that you've got ten pounds of excess for every quarter inch you pinch.

One of the keys to altering your Body Mass Index (BMI) is to get moving. See why I say exercise is truly at the heart of any weight loss program?

Another important reminder: Drink plenty of water as you work out. If you drink *at least* eight eight-ounce glasses of water a day, you'll be sure that you flush toxins from your system. I'm talking about that "metabolic garbage"—metabolized fat and toxins resulting from the calories your body consumes.

As I began my weight loss program, I got in the habit of drinking a gallon bottle of water per day. I recommend it highly. If you consume a sufficient amount of water, you will also rehydrate you body.

The human body is approximately 50 percent water. Every day, we lose about two liters of water—up to four pints—through perspiration, urination, bowel movements, and even exhalation, so, to stay healthy, we need to be aware of replacing lost bodily fluids. Much of the food we eat contains water, but usually it's not enough to replace what we expend.

Now, don't think that, because you drink a gallon of soda, a quart of milk, and "lots" of juice and other liquids during the day that you will get the benefits of pure water.

Water is water. As soon as you put something in it, it becomes something else. Caffeine, which is found in coffee, tea, and many colas, will stimulate your nervous system and make you feel energized, but it also has a diuretic effect, causing frequent urination. Milk and juices contain nutrients, and they also contain calories that you'll need to calculate into your food plan.

You can have the occasional club soda or seltzer water for variety. Some of the flavored seltzers have no calories, carbs, or fat, and they can be quite refreshing.

We've already talked about setting weight-loss goals. Now, let's look at setting a few exercise goals.

- **Keep your exercise goals realistic.** I'm not saying you should give
  yourself a pass, wimp out, and set a goal that is so reasonable a

couch potato could make it. Say that you'll do ten minutes of exercise three days a week and then do it. Anyone can do that much. You could walk from one end of the mall and back or go up and down the stairs in your house or school ten or twelve times a day, and you've met your exercise goal without setting foot in a gym.

And don't start out saying you're going to work out every single day either. Get real! If you've spent the past two years trying to figure out how to get out of gym class, there's no way on this planet that you'll suddenly start hopping out of bed and running to the gym every morning before class.

- **Make your goals specific and measurable.** To say "I'm going to exercise four times a week" is not enough. What kind of exercise are you going to do? How long will you exercise per session? How many repetitions of each exercise will you do?

  The amount of time you will exercise is measurable and so is declaring a goal of when and what time you will exercise. A specific and measurable exercise goal might be to run three miles on the treadmill in half an hour every Monday, Wednesday, and Friday. That's an admirable speed, since top Olympic distance runners run a mile in four to five minutes, so they would average six miles or so per half hour. You might decide that you will also work with free weights and do abdominal exercises for a half hour every Tuesday, Thursday, and Saturday.

  Now, if you've never been on a treadmill in your life and the closest thing to running since you were five was to come in from the rain, this goal is probably unrealistic. If that's the case, you might want to set some mini-goals, or milestones, for you to accomplish on your way to reaching your goal.

To make this happen, I recommend doing what we do with your weight-loss goals: create milestones or interim goals to keep you headed in the right direction.

For example, you might make running three miles in an hour your *long-term goal.* Then calculate how long it will take you to work up to this distance. Notice that we're not talking about setting a goal to reach a certain speed here. Not everyone can run fast, no matter how fit they are. Instead our target is distance and endurance. Once you have built up your strength and stamina, *then* you can work to increase your speed if you want.

Find out what your original ability is—say it's roughly half a mile per hour—and then project an intermediate goal that you'll increase that distance by a certain amount per week. Write down that milestone—including the date you plan to pass it (your "by when" date). This might be three-quarters of a mile per hour in one week; then one mile per hour after one more week, etc. Make up your own game.

Continue looking forward to your long-term goal, and calculate your possible rate of progress. Could you increase your speed by a half a mile per hour per week? Challenge yourself without causing injury. It's your game, so you get to make up the rules. You are not competing against anyone else. You're the only one who can win or lose.

A reminder: Neither your long-term nor interim goals are engraved in stone, and, if you fail to reach one according to your projected timetable, step back, and consider why you set them. Remember it's vital that you keep your goals realistic, not reasonable. (*Reasonable* goals aren't a challenge are they? Anyone can set goals they can reach in their sleep!)

- **Get a buddy who will hold you to your long-term goal and for the milestones on the way.** If you're the only one who knows what you're up to, who's going to hold you accountable for what you said you would do? If no one else is aware of what you're up to, who's to say you won't "forget" you've set this long-term goal six or eight weeks down the road? After a couple of weeks, when you get bored or tired and slack off, who's to know? By the end of week three, when you've given up on it altogether, who's going to kick you in the butt to get you going again? However, if you know that someone you trust is going to ask you how far and how long you're running every time he sees you, odds are you'll keep moving, and you'll keep it fun! Just pick a partner who's going to call you on your stuff when he catches you slacking off, not someone who's going to cut you some slack and allow you an easy pass.

  I know that works for me. I have my brothers, among others, to keep me honest and on target. While they haven't exactly said anything to me about it, I've been noticing that both John and Carmine have been more conscious about their own exercise habits.

If an all-out aerobic exercise program is too much for you—and it might be, if the last time you really exercised on a regular basis was the summer after third grade when you went to sleep-away camp—start out with something easier than running around the track or cross-country through your neighborhood. Find out about developing a low-impact or no-impact program. Repeated jumping and bouncing can be damaging to bones and tendons. This is especially true if you are very overweight.

Less intense, low-impact exercises are not nearly so shocking to your body. Your feet stay close to the floor, and there's one foot on the floor at all times. There's only moderate jumping around and almost no jerky, robotic movements.

No-impact aerobics call for absolutely no jumping, relying on leg lifts and other moves that exercise the large muscles of your thighs rather than those in your calves and feet. No-impact exercise calls for a lot of upper body and arm movement to start things pumping.

If low-impact calisthenics aren't for you, consider jumping on a stationary bicycle, treadmill, or elliptical machine. Most health clubs have these pieces equipment for you to use. And if your parents have 'em, all the better—especially if they've been using them as clothes racks. Just ask if you can move the bike—or NordicTrack—into your room or perhaps the family room, so you can have access to it. Your dedication to getting fit just might inspire your couch-potato parents to get moving themselves.

Another way to guarantee that you will stick to your exercise program is to choose several aerobic activities that you enjoy doing and combine this with a regular program of weight training.

What if your only aerobic exercise is playing racquet ball or tennis one afternoon a week after school, but the friend you usually play with is down with the flu, what are you going to do? Go home until your buddy's off the sick list? That's why it's important to make sure you have a Plan B in place to fall back on. So you can't play tennis today, take a few laps around the track. Or go down to the Y, and swim a few laps in the pool. Just have a backup plan so that you don't have a setback.

When you integrate your aerobic exercise with weight training, you can vary your program so that you never get bored and so that you get a total body workout.

START OUT WITH A SIMPLE WARM-UP

No matter what exercise you plan to do, take care to start out any workout session with a warm-up—four or five minutes of light activity, such as marching or jogging in place. This literally warms up your muscles. It elevates your heart rate and respiration, leaving you sweating ever so lightly.

Then do a few slow and easy stretches to lengthen your muscles: Drop you arms to your sides and lean to the left and then to the right; rotate your hips in a wide figure eight. Roll your shoulders forward, then reverse, and roll them to the back. Then stand with one foot in front of the other. Step back with one foot and lean forward into the wall to stretch your calves and hamstrings.

COOL DOWN, TOO

The reverse of warming up, a five-minute cool-down allows your heart rate to slow down gradually, so end every workout session, whether it's aerobic or purely anaerobic, with a cool-down. Slowly walk for another five minutes to lower your pulse and respiration. And since your muscles are warm and lose, stretch a bit—raise your arms over your head and then reach one arm and then the other as far up as you can; lean first to one side and then to the other, reaching your left arm over your head to the right and vice versa. Jog in place for four or five minutes.

When you cool down, you also reduce the build-up of lactic acid in your muscles. This is important because, if you don't, you'll surely be stiff, and you'll be prone to cramping. Who wants to wake up in the middle of the night with a charley horse? I don't.

Your warm-up and cool-down do not count as part of your regular exercise session. They're two distinct and important parts of your three-part exercise program.

Because if you get achy and stiff, you'll probably quit working out before you start to see any results. And you won't see any dramatic results until you've been exercising regularly for about three months, so don't give up before the miracle occurs.

PICK YOUR AEROBIC EXERCISE PLAN

I'm not going to recommend a specific aerobic-exercise program. Personally, I play lacrosse at school three or four times a week during the season and basketball, whenever the mood hits, all year long. There's nothing like a *pick-up* game or even a half hour of running the court and shooting hoops to get the heart pumping. My brothers and I, along with our friends who hang out at our house, often rev up a football or baseball game, and, as I've already said, I often take my bike out for an early morning cross-country ride.

Whatever you choose to do, just make certain that, whatever you decide to do, it's fun. It's entirely up to you to decide for yourself exactly what you can and will do. And then do it *at least* twice a week, preferably three times.

If you're clueless about what will give you the best results—and what's good for the condition of your body when you start—talk to your coach or gym teacher. If that's impossible, ask your parents to enroll you in a fitness program at the local Y or at a gym or fitness center near your home. It should be a place that offers programs specifically for teens. It needs to be accessible—a place you can go to and from without a lot of trouble, a place you feel comfortable.

You don't need to make a lifetime commitment to an expensive membership either. Start out with a three-month trial membership if possible. Then work with a trainer to evaluate the condition of your body, and design a balanced exercise program of aerobic exercise and strength training that's suited to your body's specific needs. Be aware of exactly how much you will be using the gym facilities before joining for a longer period of time.

Here's a rundown of some of the possible aerobic activities you might incorporate into your personal exercise program.

AEROBIC EXERCISE PROFILE

ACTIVITY	BENEFITS	SKILL REQUIRED
Biking	Great for aerobic conditioning, leg and arm strength, and balance.	A bit of eye-body coordination. Even if you haven't ridden a bike since fourth grade, it should come back to you. Be sure to stretch your shoulders, back, and legs before and after each ride.
Walking, Running, Jogging	Walking is the easiest and most natural of all exercise. Walking is good for cardio fitness; Running and jogging burn more calories.	Shoes designed for the sport—walking shoes are constructed differently than running shoes. Make sure they fit properly. You'll need to work up to running and/or jogging any distance.

ACTIVITY	BENEFITS	SKILL REQUIRED
Swimming*	A well-rounded form of exercise, swimming combines aerobics with strength training, all without stressing your muscles and joints.	You need a pool, and you need to know how to swim. Many health clubs and Ys have indoor pools, so you can swim all year long.
Hip-Hop Dancing	Listening to the music and moving to the beat is a great calorie-burner. In addition to boosting your heart rate and respiration, it's great for your coordination, and it's fun.	All it takes is a good CD or hot radio station. And, if hop-hop's not your bag, get moving to any music you do like.

Now list some activities *you* enjoy and get moving!

*If you're not a swimmer, call your local branch of the American Red Cross and find out where you can take swimming lessons. You might also check out water-aerobic classes. You don't have to know how to swim to get the benefits of these aerobic exercises designed for working out in the pool.

ARE YOUR BONES FULLY GROWN?

A word of warning from New York sports medicine specialist Dr. Daniel Hamner: By the time we hit our teens, we may—or may not—be fully grown. So, when you begin your diet and exercise program, ask your doctor what he or she thinks. There's a special kind of X-ray that can determine if the growth plates—the area of growing tissue near the ends of the "long bones" in children and adolescents—are closed. Also called epiphyseal plates, these plates are located at the ends of the femur, tibia, and fibula in your legs and the humerus, radius, and ulna in your arms and determine the future length and shape of the mature bone.

When we are fully grown and are as tall as we're going to be, these growth plates close and are replaced by solid bone. Until then, these plates are still fragile.

Growth plate injuries in teens and children can cause problems with bone development and growth. That's why we need to do everything possible to avoid them.

Dr. Hamner, who treats injuries for all sorts of athletes, both amateurs and pros, and is a ranked marathon runner himself, has seen just about every sports injury imaginable in his New York City practice. He says that most growth-plate injuries in teens occur during competitive sports—especially football and hockey. Basketball, soccer, tennis, baseball, and my sport, lacrosse, involve less physical contact and are less likely to cause such serious injury. (I know. I know. Lacrosse can get vicious, but in reality, it's not a contact sport like football, ice hockey, and rugby.)

If you are injured while playing a sport or doing any kind of exercise, especially if it affects your athletic performance or your ability to move or put pressure on a limb, head for the doctor. You should never, ever be allowed—or expected—to work through the pain.

You may experience some discomfort—muscle cramps, stiffness, and such—as you learn new skills, but if this discomfort doesn't go away or becomes painful, get to the doctor. If you don't have it taken care of, some injuries can cause permanent damage and interfere with bone growth.

EXERCISES I DO TO STAY FIT

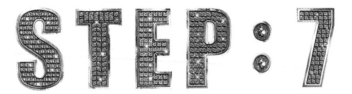

STEP : 7

LIFT EXTRA POUNDS, DON'T GAIN THEM

Two years ago, when I started my personal quest for weight loss and fitness, I never dreamed I could have a cut and toned body. I can finally see my neck! No problem!

I just decided not to be fat anymore, and I got tired of the teasing and name-calling.

When I was still fat, I played basketball and lacrosse at school—but even that wasn't enough exercise for me to be able to lose weight. Looking back, I hate to admit it, but as athletic as I have always been, it really was difficult to run up and down the court or across the lacrosse field when I weighed more than 250 pounds.

I was never able to do one pull-up, not one. I remember how I would look at the bar and just *wish* I could do one. Even the skinny, nonathletic kids who stunk at sports could do one.

I didn't notice that at the time, that's just the way it was: I couldn't run far or fast. But now, as I look back, it was physically exhausting for me to be lugging around all those extra pounds. And, if you're anything at all like me, you probably eat more when you're overly tired. And you'll probably reach for something sweet in hopes of getting that energy-boosting sugar rush you feel you need.

The amazing thing I have learned is that it is protein—like a piece of cheese or a couple of slices of turkey—that raises my energy level more than a candy bar or bowl of ice cream. High sugar carbohydrates are what are called high glycemic foods, which means they are quickly turned into sugar. They may give you a quick energy boost, but they also make you crash just as quickly.

Within a few weeks of adding weight training to my overall exercise regimen, I found myself looking forward to my workout sessions. I had more energy; I felt stronger, and I quickly began to experience a definite increase in energy. The pounds began to go.

Within three months, I saw definition in my shoulders, arms, torso, and legs. Yet I wasn't bulking up too much either.

So, this leads me to the final step of my *7 Steps for Healthy Weight Loss For Teens.*

STEP 7: LIFT EXTRA POUNDS, DON'T GAIN THEM

Lifting weights will not, I repeat not, turn you into a muscle-bound hulk, unless of course you want it to, and then, only if you're fully grown. However, weight lifting will enable you to build lean body mass, using moderate weights to do a few very simple exercises, to develop well-defined, cut muscles. That *is* what you want, isn't it?

Let me stress the word *moderate*. There is a major debate among doctors and educators about the use of weights before your skeletal system has finished growing. Generally speaking, this last great growth spurt starts around age twelve and ends at seventeen or eighteen, but some of us shoot up fast and stop growing at a younger age. I did. I was six-one by the time I hit fourteen. Looking at my family, I could tell that, in all probability, I would not be growing much taller.

Your doctor can do a special X-ray of the back of your hip bones to see if the growth plates at the ends of your long bones have closed. Another test—another kind of X-ray—can determine your bone density if there are any questions about the strength of your bones.

Dr. Hamner suggests that, if you plan to work out on machines, start out by working with a trainer—especially if you're not certain that you have reached your full height and body size. A qualified trainer will be able to determine if you are physically ready to work with weights and other pieces of gym equipment and can instruct you in how to work with it so that you are not injured.

For example, when doing leg extensions, you might decide to use ankle weights or add weight to the machines, but don't do it without the advice of an expert. If you add too much weight, you could damage the growth plates at the bottom of your knees, actually dislodging them. This is painful and potentially permanently damaging.

If there is any doubt if you are physically mature enough to work with the equipment, the trainer or facility manager may refuse to permit you to work out with the equipment without a physical exam and written permission from your doctor.

Do not get all macho, and shop around for another gym until you get your way. That's asking for big trouble and a lot of pain. Only an irresponsible trainer or facility will allow someone whose body is not fully mature to do exercises that are potentially dangerous. Remember that, and remember that when your body is ready for weight work, it will respond with great results.

As Dr. Hamner has warned, the danger in weight work before you have stopped growing lies in the fact that you risk serious and even permanent injury.

FIND A BALANCE BETWEEN DIET AND EXERCISE

Exercise, together with a balanced diet for weight loss not only strengthens your muscles, it also keeps your skin taut and toned. Your skin has been stretched by your excess fat like when you blow up a balloon. While exercising aerobically will burn fat, anaerobic exercise, such as weight training, pull-ups, sit-ups, and push-ups, will develop strength and lean muscle mass which provides a fit and firm foundation for your skin.

If you lose weight too quickly, your skin can become loose and rippled, kind of like what happens when you let the air out of a balloon. Without a lean, muscular form to give it shape, you'll look worn and wrinkled, even if you're still in your teens.

Weight training has helped me develop endurance strength, which is the basis of overall strength. The bonus is that my weight loss and newfound endurance have made me better at the performance sports I enjoy. I can run faster and longer without huffing and puffing; I can throw farther; twist and turn easily; and jump, roll, and spin without hurting myself. It's an awesome feeling. I have trimmed my weight down, developed a lean body, and increased my energy level and stamina beyond anything I dared hope.

Anaerobic exercise, such as weight lifting, involves short spurts of exertion, followed by rest. The results are better muscle definition, endurance, and strength. With this as a base, you will be better prepared for sports that combine aerobic and anaerobic exercise, like basketball, lacrosse, and field hockey, as well as for a purely aerobic exercise like long distance running.

Weight training, also known as resistance training, completes the process, building lean body mass, and improving bone strength, muscle joints, and connective tissue.

But a program that is solely aerobic or solely anaerobic is not enough for weight loss. A lean, toned body burns calories more efficiently than one that is fleshy and fat. In fact, ACSM studies indicate that weight training burns calories even after you've quit working out. This indicates that resistance training, which builds lean muscle mass, is just as important as aerobic exercise, which consumes calories by elevating your heart rate and respiration, to form a complete weight-loss program. For a well-rounded weight-loss and fitness program, you've got to do both.

Aerobic exercise is characterized by increased breathing and an elevated heart rate over an extended period of time. After about ten minutes of an aerobic workout, your body starts burning up its stored fat reserves as fuel.

The muscle-building results of an anaerobic program complement aerobic exercise and enable you to perform more skillfully. Your larger muscles will burn more calories during exercise too.

BEFORE YOU LIFT THAT FIRST WEIGHT

Dr. Hamner says that how much weight you can lift is not nearly as important as how many reps you can do. A good target for any exercise is three sets of twenty to twenty-five reps with fifteen- to twenty-pound free weights.

Start with five- or ten-pound dumbbells, whichever you can lift comfortably—especially if you've never done weight training before. Don't try to show off, and start out working with twenty-pound weights or bench pressing sixty pounds on your first try. You can get hurt that way.

You can even start with three- or four-pound free weights if there is any possibility that you could injure yourself. Trust your gut. It's nobody else's business about how much weight you're pressing.

A school friend who had been battling his weight as I had told me he wanted to do what I was doing—lose weight—and said that he was going to start pumping iron. One day after school he stopped by our house, and we started talking about exercise. He said he was going to start lifting weights with his older brothers, so he could get cut and buff.

I warned him to take it easy and start out slowly and started to explain why that is important, but he said he was strong enough and wouldn't listen to what I was saying, even when Mom told him that I was right.

A couple of weeks later I heard that his mother had taken him to the doctor because he had started to have intense chest pains.

As he began to examine my friend, the doctor immediately asked if he had been working with weights.

His mom said, "Oh no, he. . . ."

My friend cut her off and confessed that indeed he had been pumping iron with his brothers.

Then I found out that he was in the hospital, having a hernia—a rip—in his pericardium, the membranous sac around his heart, repaired. I don't know how much weight he was pressing, but it was enough to cause serious damage to his heart.

If his doctor hadn't been aware that this particular type of injury could happen from lifting too much weight, my friend could have *died*.

GETTING STARTED

Once you've done five minutes or so of aerobic, warm-up exercise—marching in place, jumping jacks, five minutes on the treadmill or a stationery bike to raise your *heart rate* and respiration, and warm up your muscles—you're ready to begin your weight training.

Start out doing three sets of twenty or twenty-five repetitions of each exercise you are including in that day's workout. The third set will be the most difficult. You'll begin to feel your muscles working hard.

Continue working with this amount of weight for as many days as you feel like your muscles are really working. When that third set starts to feel as easy as your first, then it's time to move up a level to heavier weights. This will happen after two or three weeks, maybe even longer.

This is important: Resist the urge to increase the *number* of reps you do. Instead, increase the *weight* you are lifting. Move up in no more than five-pound increments. For instance, go from five-pound weights to ten-pound weights, then from ten-pound weights to fifteen-pounders, and keep on working.

Following this formula of three sets of twenty to twenty-five lifts until all three sets feel too easy, increase the weight you lift in five-pound increments until you are working with twenty-five-pound weights.

Dr. Hamner and other experts recommend that those of us who're under eighteen stick with twenty-five-pound weights to maintain muscle tone and form.

That's okay. Right now I just want to be fit and firm; I'm not training to become Mr. Universe.

VARY YOUR WORKOUT ROUTINE

I don't do the same exercises every day, but I do work out daily. By varying my program, I don't get bored, and I don't concentrate on any one muscle group. One day, I might concentrate on my biceps, triceps, and pecs; the next I'll work on my lats and upper abdomen. One day it may be pull-ups and sit-ups, and then push-ups and crunches the next.

Remember:

- Develop an exercise routine that works for you, and then work at it at your own pace.

- Compete with yourself, not with someone else. Save the competition for team sports. NOTE: This doesn't mean you have to exercise alone. It's always fun to have workout partners to keep you honest!

- Make beating your personal best your quest. Keep your eye on that prize.

- Keep track of your progress.

What is important is that you do *some* exercise on a regular basis. After all, *some is better than none*. Start out doing as many reps as you can per exercise and increase as you build strength. Don't worry if you can only do one set of ten curls with five-pound weights and only two pull-ups when you start out. You will get better at it.

Remember the grief you got in phys-ed class when you couldn't pull yourself up the rope or when you could barely make it around the track when Coach had everybody running laps? Build endurance strength, and you will never be embarrassed like that again.

When I started out, I wasn't able to do one pull-up. I remember that I used to look up at that bar and wish I could do just one. Now that I have lost all my weight, I can do, like, ten, no problem. I feel like I have way more stamina than I did when I was fat.

SQUAT, WALK, JUMP, AND CRUNCH TO THE BEAT

I always exercise to music. It keeps my energy up—big time. I'm a big fan of hip-hop—Jadakiss, Fat Joe, The Game, G-Unit, Camron—and keep a stack of CDs handy whenever I start a workout session. You might say this is my feel-good music.

However, before you start downloading tunes into your iPod, let me give you a word of warning about working out with music: Don't exercise *to* the music. Concentrate on the rhythm of your exercise and *not* the beat of the band. If you catch yourself doing biceps curls to a hip-hop beat, change your pace.

Control your muscles as you exercise. Concentrate on the muscle groups that you are working, and keep your movements slow and steady.

Starting position for standing exercises:

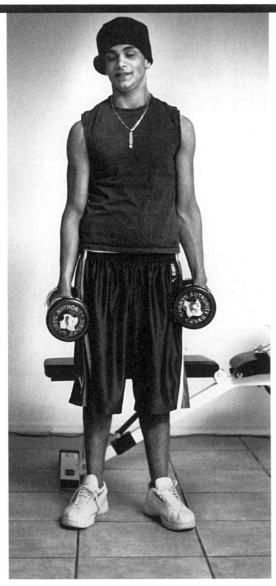

Stand erect with your feet hip-width apart. Keep your knees loose and relaxed, arms hanging loosely at your side, palms parallel with your body. Hold one weight in each hand. Keep your wrists, palms, and fingers relaxed. Do not hold weights with a death grip. Your hands will cramp—not good.

STANDING ALTERNATE CURLS

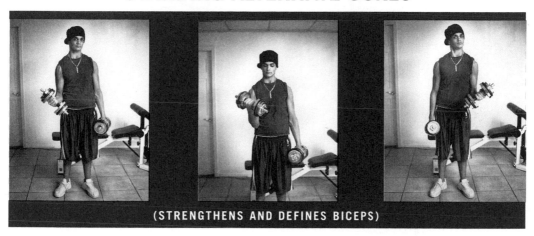

(STRENGTHENS AND DEFINES BICEPS)

From the basic starting position, hold weights parallel to your hips. Curl one arm up, bringing that hand to shoulder level, rotating your hands so that your palms face your chest, and weights are parallel to your chest. Control movement as you return to the starting position. Alternate arms. Goal: three sets of twenty to twenty-five reps.

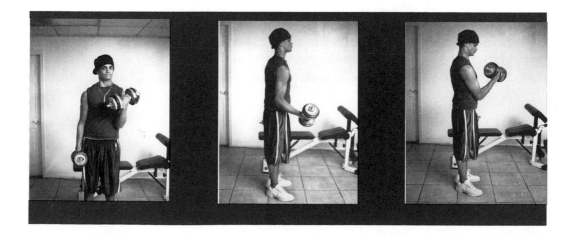

FRONT LATERAL LIFTS

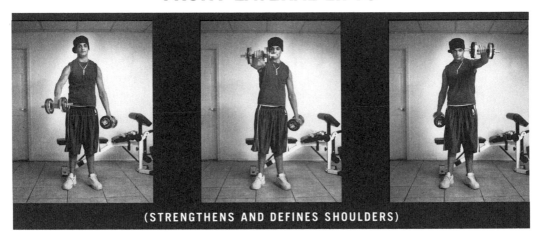

(STRENGTHENS AND DEFINES SHOULDERS)

From the basic starting position, lift right arm to shoulder level in front of your body. Keep your elbows soft, and rotate hands down, holding weights parallel to the floor. Control the movement as you lower your arm to the starting position. Alternate arms. Goal: three sets of twenty to twenty-five reps.

ALTERNATING ARM PRESS

(STRENGTHENS AND DEFINES BICEPS)

From the basic starting position, stand straight with arms bent and weights held at shoulder level. Lift one arm straight up over your head until arm is straight. Do not lock your elbows. Control your movement as you return to your original position. Alternate right arm and left arm. Goal: three sets of twenty to twenty-five reps.

HORIZONTAL SHOULDER EXERCISES

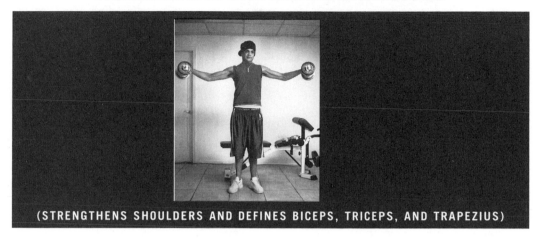

(STRENGTHENS SHOULDERS AND DEFINES BICEPS, TRICEPS, AND TRAPEZIUS)

From basic starting position, slowly lift both arms out to the side, raising them to shoulder level. Keep elbows soft and your palms turned downward. Control movement as you lower your arm to the starting position. Goal: three sets of twenty to twenty-five reps.

NOTE: You can lift one arm at a time, alternating from right to left, or lift both arms at the same time, whichever feels most comfortable to you. The power of this exercise is in the control of your movements up and down.

HORIZONTAL LIFTS

(STRENGTHENS SHOULDERS, DEFINES BICEPS AND TRICEPS, AND STRETCHES TRAPEZIUS)

From basic starting position with your legs no more than hip-width apart, lean forward from the waist. Keep your knees loose and relaxed. With your arms hanging toward the floor at shoulder width, hold weights down, parallel to your legs. Keep knees slightly bent and elbows relaxed. Lift arms out to each side, and slowly lower arms back to the starting position. Goal: three sets of twenty to twenty-five reps.

Basic Starting Position for Kneeling-Bench Exercises:

Standing to the side of a bench or sturdy chair, place one knee on the bench and lean forward, stabilizing your body by placing your hand firmly on the seat. (For instance, if you place your left knee on the bench, put your left hand on the seat.) Move other leg, slightly bent, to the rear. Hold weight in your other hand, keeping your arm relaxed toward the floor. When you complete your targeted number of sets and reps for this position, move to the other side of the bench, and then exercise using your other hand and arm.

TRICEP CURLS

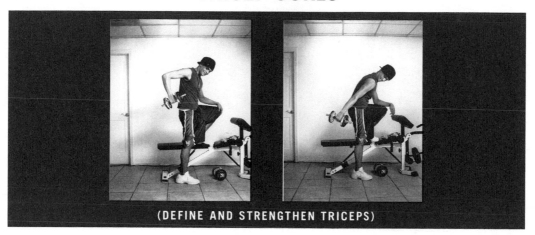

(DEFINE AND STRENGTHEN TRICEPS)

From the basic starting position for kneeling-bench exercises, slowly lift your outside elbow, and lift the weight to shoulder level, rotating your wrist so that the palm is up. Then
extend arm back to a horizontal position parallel to your back and control movement as
you return to the starting position. Switch arms and repeat, kneeling on your left knee
and working the weight with your right arm. Goal: three sets of twenty to twenty-five reps,
each arm.

TRIANGLE CURLS

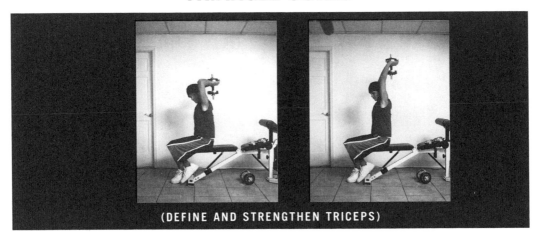

(DEFINE AND STRENGTHEN TRICEPS)

Sitting on a chair or bench, grasp one dumbbell, vertically, with both hands at the top end. Hold it with the weights in your palms, not by the handle. Raise arms to the ceiling, holding the weight over your head. Control your movement as you lower the weight behind your head. Keep your back straight, and hold your head erect so that you are facing forward. Repeat. Goal: three sets of twenty to twenty-five reps.

VARIATION: Lie with your back flat on the bench, and do the exercise from that position. Take care that you keep your arms relaxed. Do not stiffen your elbows.

PULL-UPS

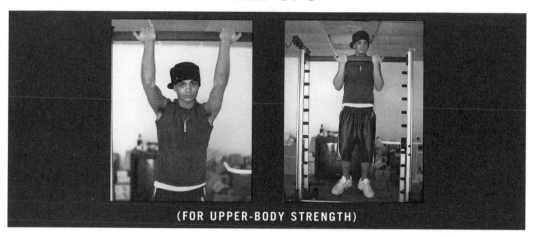

(FOR UPPER-BODY STRENGTH)

Reach over your head, and grasp a chinning bar with both hands, palms *forward*. Position hands at shoulder width, and grasp the bar. Pull yourself up, like you were going to chin yourself on the bar. Control your movement as you lift, and lower your body. Start by doing as many pull-ups as you can. Goal: three sets of twenty.

ONE ARM SAWING

(STRENGTHENS AND DEFINES BICEPS)

From starting position, leaning forward hold weight in your left (outside) hand. Keeping arm relaxed and straight downward, bend your elbow, and lift weight to your chest. Keeping your upper arm close to your rib cage, parallel to your back, move arm in a back and forth sawing motion. Control movement as you lower your arm. Switch arms, and repeat, using your right arm. Goal: three sets of twenty to twenty-five reps each arm.

CHIN-UPS

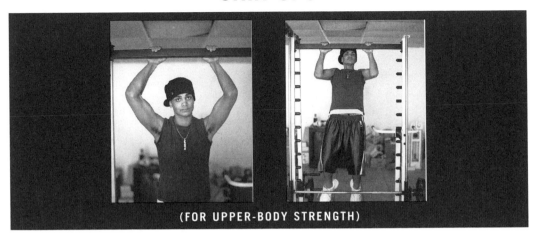

(FOR UPPER-BODY STRENGTH)

Reach over your head, and grasp a chinning bar with both hands, palms *away from your face.* Position hands at shoulder width, and grasp the bar. Pull your body up, to chin yourself on the bar. Control your movement as you lift and lower your body. Start by doing as many pull-ups as you can. Goal: three sets of twenty.

NOTE: According to Dr. Hamner, pull-ups and chin-ups are "the best exercise ever" for the upper body, affecting the triceps, all of the deltoids, the lats, all back and chest muscles, the radius anterior, and the upper abdominals. The trouble is, if you're especially heavy, you may not be able to do either, yet. Keep working. Before long, you will be able to both pull-ups and chin-ups. Dr. Hamner says that push-ups, which everyone knows how to do, run a distant second in building strength.

PUSH-UPS

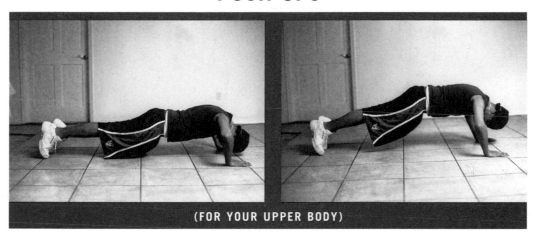

(FOR YOUR UPPER BODY)

Lying prone on an exercise mat, position hands on the floor, shoulder width apart. Bend your knees, lifting your feet from the floor. Push your upper body away from the floor until arms are straight. Do not lock your elbows. Control your movement as you lower your body almost to the floor; straighten arms to lift again. Start by doing as many push-ups as you can. Goal: three sets of twenty-five.

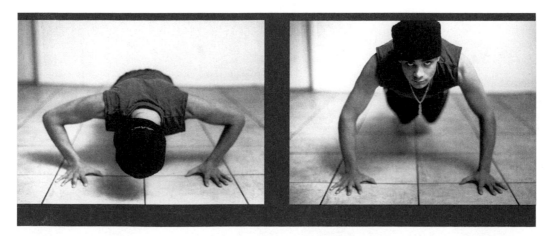

SIT-UPS

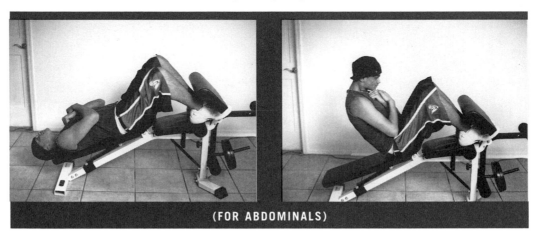

(FOR ABDOMINALS)

Start out on the floor or a mat. As you become stronger, you can do your sit-ups and crunches on a slant. (See variation below.)

Anchor your feet under a strap, or, as I do when I'm not working out on the bench, under the couch. You can also have a friend hold your feet down. Lie back with your knees bent. Cross your arms loosely across your chest, and lift your shoulders from the floor as

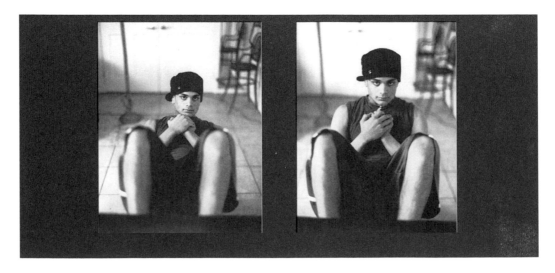

you tighten your upper-abdominal muscles to curl your upper body upward. Control your movement, and roll back to starting position. Lower abs support your lower back and legs. Dr. Hamner recommends that as you start working out, place your palms on your lower abdomen so that you will be able to get feedback on how you are contracting your abdominal muscles as you exercise. Goal: three sets of twenty-five.

IMPORTANT NOTE: You may have been doing sit-ups with your hands behind your head. *Never* place your fingers behind your neck or pull your upper body upward from that position. If you do, you're risking injury to your neck.

VARIATION: I frequently add resistance to my sit-ups by asking someone to stand above me and push my shoulders back down as I am moving upward. If no one is available to help you out, you can set the bench on an angle, so you're doing your sit-ups (or crunches) uphill for extra resistance, as I'm demonstrating here.

CRUNCHES

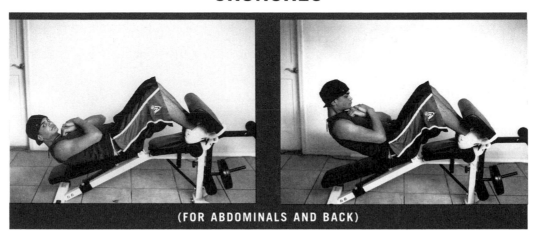

(FOR ABDOMINALS AND BACK)

Lying on your back, pull your knees to your chest, keeping your legs relaxed. Place your hands behind your head. Curl your upper body off the floor toward your knees. Do *not* pull your head up with your arms, and do not rock back and forth to lift body. Control your movement up and back to the starting position. Again, I'm working on a slanted board. As you grow stronger and have access to a weight bench, you might give this version a try too. Goal: three sets of twenty-five.

TRACKING YOUR OWN SUCCESS

RECORDING YOUR WEIGHT-LOSS, FOOD,

AND FITNESS PLAN

Use the charts in this chapter to document and track your personal progress as you begin your 7-Step Program to lose weight and get in shape. By putting this information down and noting your observations on paper, you will be better able to keep your program in action.

Vital Statistics

STARTING WEIGHT: _____

TARGET WEIGHT: _____

DATE: _____

BY WHEN: _____

After 1 Month: _____

After 2 Months: _____

After 3 Months: _____

After 4 Months: _____

After 5 Months: _____

After 6 Months: _____

After 7 Months: _____

After 8 Months: _____

After 9 Months: _____

After 10 Months: _____

After 11 Months: _____

After 12 Months: _____

As a very wise man once said, you'll never know when you've arrived unless you know where you're going.

To get a handle on your eating habits, keep a food journal every day for at least a week. Remember to look for any patterns you may see here. Do you eat seconds at every meal? Do you skip the green vegetables and salads for potatoes and gravy or mac and cheese? Be honest with yourself.

DAILY FOOD JOURNAL

DATE_____

WHEN AND WHERE I ATE	WHAT I ATE . . . AND HOW MUCH	WHAT I WAS FEELING OR DOING

A suggestion: Photocopy this form, and repeat this Daily Food Journal process every few months to raise your awareness of how and what you are eating—how your eating habits are changing.

You may also want to keep a diary of your foods as you begin to eliminate foods you don't want to eat because they cause weight gain. Again, this will keep you in touch with when and what you're eating.

As you work out, log your progress on the following charts. I recommend copying these pages—one per exercise per week—so you can watch your progress.

Notice that I haven't given you a page for the starting positions—they're part of the exercises—and I haven't given you a journal to write about your aerobic activity. You're on your honor to make sure you fit true aerobic exercise into your weight-loss and fitness program.

WEIGHT AND STRENGTH TRAINING

Alternating Arm Press

(STRENGTHENS AND DEFINES BICEPS)

WEEK #: _____

DATES: _____

WEIGHT USED: _____

DAY	SETS DONE	REPS PER SET	NOTES
Monday			
Tuesday			
Wednesday			
Thursday			
Friday			
Saturday			
Sunday			

Standing Alternate Curls

(STRENGTHENS AND DEFINES BICEPS)

WEEK #: _____

DATES: _____

WEIGHT USED: _____

DAY	SETS DONE	REPS PER SET	NOTES
Monday			
Tuesday			
Wednesday			
Thursday			
Friday			
Saturday			
Sunday			

Front Lateral Press

(STRENGTHENS AND DEFINES TRICEPS)

WEEK #: _____

DATES: _____

WEIGHT USED: _____

DAY	SETS DONE	REPS PER SET	NOTES
Monday			
Tuesday			
Wednesday			
Thursday			
Friday			
Saturday			
Sunday			

Front Lateral Lift

(STRENGTHENS AND DEFINES SHOULDERS)

WEEK #: _____

DATES: _____

WEIGHT USED: _____

DAY	SETS DONE	REPS PER SET	NOTES
Monday			
Tuesday			
Wednesday			
Thursday			
Friday			
Saturday			
Sunday			

Horizontal Shoulder Exercises

(STRENGTHEN SHOULDERS, DEFINES BICEPS, TRICEPS, AND TRAPEZIUS)

WEEK #: _____

DATES: _____

WEIGHT USED: _____

DAY	SETS DONE	REPS PER SET	NOTES
Monday			
Tuesday			
Wednesday			
Thursday			
Friday			
Saturday			
Sunday			

Horizontal Lifts

(STRENGTHEN SHOULDERS, DEFINES BICEPS, AND TRICEPS AND STRETCHES TRAPEZIUS)

WEEK #: _____

DATES: _____

WEIGHT USED: _____

DAY	SETS DONE	REPS PER SET	NOTES
Monday			
Tuesday			
Wednesday			
Thursday			
Friday			
Saturday			
Sunday			

Tricep Curls

(DEFINES AND STRENGTHENS TRICEPS)

WEEK #: _____

DATES: _____

WEIGHT USED: _____

DAY	SETS DONE	REPS PER SET	NOTES
Monday			
Tuesday			
Wednesday			
Thursday			
Friday			
Saturday			
Sunday			

Triangle Curls

(DEFINES AND STRENGTHENS TRICEPS)

WEEK #: _____

DATES: _____

WEIGHT USED: _____

DAY	SETS DONE	REPS PER SET	NOTES
Monday			
Tuesday			
Wednesday			
Thursday			
Friday			
Saturday			
Sunday			

One Arm Sawing

(STRENGTHENS BICEPS AND TRICEPS)

WEEK #: _____

DATES: _____

WEIGHT USED: _____

DAY	SETS DONE	REPS PER SET	NOTES
Monday			
Tuesday			
Wednesday			
Thursday			
Friday			
Saturday			
Sunday			

Pull-Ups

(FOR UPPER-BODY STRENGTH)

WEEK #: _____

DATES: _____

DAY	SETS DONE	REPS PER SET	NOTES
Monday			
Tuesday			
Wednesday			
Thursday			
Friday			
Saturday			
Sunday			

Chin-Ups

(FOR UPPER-BODY STRENGTH)

WEEK #: _____

DATES: _____

DAY	SETS DONE	REPS PER SET	NOTES
Monday			
Tuesday			
Wednesday			
Thursday			
Friday			
Saturday			
Sunday			

Push-Ups

(FOR UPPER-BODY STRENGTH)

WEEK #: _____

DATES: _____

DAY	SETS DONE	REPS PER SET	NOTES
Monday			
Tuesday			
Wednesday			
Thursday			
Friday			
Saturday			
Sunday			

Sit-Ups

(FOR ABDOMINALS)

WEEK #: _____

DATES: _____

DAY	SETS DONE	REPS PER SET	NOTES
Monday			
Tuesday			
Wednesday			
Thursday			
Friday			
Saturday			
Sunday			

Sit-Ups Variation

(FOR ABDOMINALS)

WEEK #: _____

DATES: _____

DAY	SETS DONE	REPS PER SET	NOTES
Monday			
Tuesday			
Wednesday			
Thursday			
Friday			
Saturday			
Sunday			

Crunches

(FOR ABDOMINALS AND BACK)

WEEK #: _____

DATES: _____

DAY	SETS DONE	REPS PER SET	NOTES
Monday			
Tuesday			
Wednesday			
Thursday			
Friday			
Saturday			
Sunday			

I CAN DO ANYTHING

THE PROOF IS IN MY BODY!

I didn't get to spend much time with my grandpa John, but I certainly learned a lot from him. My parents and grandma Victoria, Sr.—as well as my aunt Angel and uncles Peter and John—made sure of that, especially making sure that my brothers and I knew his views about some very important life lessons—like how we could do anything we set our minds to.

"You can do whatever you want, you can be anybody you want to be, but nobody can do it for you." That's what he said.

Okay, so I could do anything I wanted, but nobody could do it for me. What I needed was a dose of discipline.

So, with Grandpa's words echoing in my head—I've been able to do just that. Good grades—I made First Honors; sports—from Little League baseball to basketball and lacrosse; I even managed to win friends—I have many. In many ways, I've led a charmed life.

But I had no self-discipline as far as my weight was concerned. Weight problem? What weight problem? I ate, I got fat, no problem.

Of course, looking back to two years ago, my weight really *was* a problem, only I wasn't facing it. I couldn't, and, as Grandpa said, nobody was going to do it for me.

I guess I thought that if I didn't talk about it, my weight didn't matter, so I kept my mouth shut. Figuratively speaking, that is.

You wouldn't catch me hanging out at the mall. I couldn't stand to go shopping for clothes. School didn't matter—we wear uniforms—but even something as seemingly simple as buying a pair of jeans or stocking up on underwear was embarrassing—an awful experience. I wouldn't do it. I wouldn't even go into the store. I let my Mom do the shopping. If something didn't fit, she could always take it back for a larger size.

One Christmas, when I told her I wanted some clothes, she asked me for my sizes. I was embarrassed to give her a specific number, so I just said, "XL, maybe XXL."

Who was I kidding?

Mom told me later she thought I wanted something loose and baggie, like all the kids my age wore.

I was too ashamed to tell her that my clothes didn't fit any more. It seemed I went up a waist size every month—thirty-six, thirty-eight, forty, forty-two, forty-four, then I hit forty-six. I couldn't even look Mom in the eye when I had to tell her that I was "a little bigger than a forty-six."

I was twelve years old.

Mom went into the Annexx Shop, where we always got our uniforms for school and everything else we wore. She told Barry, the salesman, what she was looking for and gave him everybody's sizes. Carmine and John, size thirty-two—medium; Frankie? "What's a little bigger than a forty-six?"

Barry, who had been helping us with our clothes for years, replied, "Beyond forty-six? Mrs. G, this is the last time, we'll be able to fit Frankie."

I wasn't interested in dressing up. To me, clothes were just material to cover my body. I did not enjoy picking out clothes one bit. And, since most of my friends were my size or not much smaller than me, well, it didn't matter how I dressed. Everything made me look fat and sloppy.

I saw the worry in my mother's eyes, but she rarely said a thing to me about how much I ate or anything like that. Oh, there was the occasional "Save some of that for your brothers," but little else.

Grandpa John, however, didn't pull any punches, but he wasn't hurtful either. "Sure you're a bit overweight, Frank, but you're the most handsome boy in the group," he told me once when my brothers and I went to visit him. "Ask your mom what I told her the day you were born. I saw you in the hospital crib through the window, and I said, 'All my grandkids are handsome as hell, but this kid has the movie star look. He's the one.'"

The concept of being good looking—never mind having "the movie star look"—escaped me at the time. But every time I saw him, Grandpa made a point of reminding me that I had been more than blessed in the looks department.

When I looked in the mirror, which didn't happen often if I could help it, I couldn't see what he was talking about. In fact, I saw a fat, sloppy-dressing kid with several flabby chins and no neck that anyone could see. I didn't like looking at him at all.

Anyone meeting me for the first time would say that I was shy, quiet, self-conscious, and fat.

Back in the day I had to struggle into XXXL sweats and stretched-out T-shirts. I really hated the idea that my family would be doing a TV show and that we would be playing ourselves. My mom is beautiful. Everyone says she's hot. And my brothers are good looking and popular, too. Carmine was class president, and everybody loves John. Girls are always flirting with them. I was their big, fat little brother.

It's no surprise that the show jump-started my desire to shape up. Fueled by this desire and the self-confidence that would came with it, I was able to discover what it would take for me to lose weight and get fit.

By the time we had the launch party for *Growing Up Gotti*, I was unrecognizable to people who had only seen me as the fat kid. In fact, I hardly recognized me either. Who was this guy in the dark, charcoal Sean John suit that was a perfect fit and the well-styled hair? At the A&E party I not only looked cool, I also *felt* cool.

Hey, I realized, I really *do* look like a TV star, and the TV cameras that follow me around prove it.

Now, I actually enjoy shopping for myself. I like to try things on and check everything out in the mirror. That's the absolute opposite of two years ago when it was hard to get me to go into a store and downright impossible to get me into a dressing room to try things on. Who can blame me? I used to be shaped like Shrek; now I have a thirty-two inch waist.

I can now walk into any store I want and find something good to wear. My favorite designers are Armani Exchange, Abercrombie & Fitch, and Sean John.

Talk about a major change in my appearance: I've even been asked to model in fashion shows!

Mom says that I have become a *fashionista*—big time. She accuses me of spending far too much time looking at myself in the full-length mirror in her bedroom.

What's wrong with that? A guy has to make sure everything looks just right before he goes out. I may have to wear a uniform to school, but my hair has to be cool. And, hey, I'm not going over to my girl's house or out with the guys looking like a slob in baggie sweats. Not now.

In addition to looking 200 percent better than I did two years ago, I have about 200 percent more energy. This is not to say I wasn't active before, but I did get tired a lot faster. Now I have an extreme amount of stamina and strength, and I finally have a neck! I can see it—no problem. That has certainly been good for my self-image.

The past year and a half of healthy eating has definitely been worth it. I have no regrets, and I have changed how I will eat, exercise, and care for my body for the rest of my life.

Another interesting outcome of my personal weight-loss campaign has been watching my friends begin to take charge of their own bodies. I had never thought of myself as a role model before!

My cousin Bobby—we're almost the same age—is watching his food intake and working out. Because he asked his mother, Susan, to support him and because he asked me to help him, he may *think* about cheating and eating junk food, but he's not getting away with it.

My friend Brian's mom called mine to tell her that she couldn't think of anyone more qualified than me to encourage Brian to lose weight. She told Mom that I'm harder on him than she is, telling Mom that I used tough love with him, that I had told Brian he has to help himself.

I really did. I told him, "You've gotta do it yourself. You've been asking me how I've done it for a year now, but you haven't done a thing about it yet. You're not going to swallow a magic pill and wake up thin. You've got to work at it."

I told him as I'm telling you: "You've got to want to lose weight for yourself and not for anyone else."

Because I had just watched Brian eat three doughnuts, I confessed, "Yo, it's difficult to be around you because I feel like you're a temptation to me."

That really caught him short. Brian and I had been pals for a long time. I don't think he thought I would every say anything so bluntly.

Another big difference between "then" and "now" is that I've come out of my shell. I'm still a little shy, a little quiet, a little reserved, but I'm not about to blow off anyone who sincerely wants to talk to me about losing weight and getting in shape.

I know what it's like to be self-conscious about my body. I remember hiding out in my bedroom and just eating. I know what it's like to see people look away when you jump into the pool with your T-shirt on.

I remember how easily I could feel lonely in a crowd, when girls were walking right past me to flirt with one of my brothers or a stranger would turn away when I stopped to introduce myself.

And I also know how painful it is when your parents talk with your teachers or your doctor about your weight as though you can't hear them when all the while you're sitting right there in front of them. We can know that it's just because they're worried about you, but that doesn't make it hurt any less.

None of that happens to me any more.

I don't just look better or feel better, but I am much more comfortable in my skin. I have confidence. Not the "Hey, look at me!" kind, but the kind that makes me feel able to handle any circumstance that comes my way. May you all feel so good.

A MOTHER'S UNCONDITIONAL LOVE

MY MOM HAS SOMETHING TO SAY

Having an overweight child is not unlike having a sickly child. Obesity becomes an all-consuming cause for concern.

With Frankie, I found myself helpless—hands tied behind my back. Every time he reached for a piece of cake or dug into a hearty bowl of pasta, I would silently reprimand him with a barrage of unsaid, unkind remarks. "Do you really need to eat all of that?" or "Doesn't he know how fattening that is?"

All the while, I studiously avoided my son's eyes for fear he would pick up on the fact that I was upset—not upset because he was eating, mind you—but because I knew he would put on more weight and soon it would affect his health.

As the mom, I was also faced with the knowledge that I could not *not* feed Frank. As large as he was, Frank was still a growing boy. I had to make sure he got all the nutrients he needed to stay healthy, but I also was faced with the fact that he was growing bigger and bigger before my very eyes.

I realize now how cruel and ridiculous all this was, especially now that I know that food became Frank's source of comfort during some terribly traumatic times for our family—like my divorce from Frank's father and his grandpa's death from cancer.

We all have a vice—something not so healthy or good for us. It could be smoking or drinking, even overeating, anything that we do as a means to escape. Frank's vice-of-choice was food, gorging himself to numb how badly he hurt inside.

Watching Frank's weight balloon hurt me even more than if I had gained the weight myself. I remember lying awake at night in tears or even pacing the floors in search of a solution. If only Frank's "condition" were as easy to cure as a general childhood illness like chicken pox, mumps, or measles. If only I could give him a tablespoon of cough syrup or a series of antibiotic pills.

I would just as soon suffer total devastation rather than see any of my sons suffer from even a miniscule toothache. Still, I couldn't figure out how to even bring up the subject of Frank's weight, let alone find a cure for his overeating and overweight.

I kept telling myself there had to be a easy method to help him shed those unhealthy pounds. He was active, he played sports, and he ate a lot.

One thing I did know was how cruel school kids could be. I could remember all too well how hurt I was when my sister Angel's classmates and playmates teased her mercilessly about her weight, and even how they made fun of me for being so skinny—"Olive Oyl!," "Pencil Legs!," "Skinny Minnie!" And let's not even talk about the names I was called because I wore glasses! They were bright blue cat's-eye glasses with rhinestones in the corners, and they made me the object of ridicule everywhere I turned.

I had suffered the cruelty of name-calling and being left out by my own classmates as I was growing up. But just imagining how kids were teasing Frank, saying unkind, even hateful things to him, tore at my heartstrings far worse than anything that had been said to me when I was a kid.

As a mom, I wanted to protect my youngest son from all bad things. Let nothing harm him. I could chase the Boogeyman and all the monsters under the bed, but how was I to know the culprits making my child's life miserable would be eight-, nine-, and ten-year-old boys and girls.

I considered having a talk with Frankie's teachers, possibly putting them on alert to any name-calling or teasing. Perhaps I would call the parents of his classmates and warn them that I would make trouble if their kids teased my son. But I realized neither was the answer and would probably serve to antagonize matters even further. I had to get to the root of the problem.

I had to figure out a way to inspire Frank to want to lose the weight himself.

For starters, I took Frank in to see his general practitioner for his regular school physical. Dr. Steve Rucker is a wonderful physician in his early forties, not yet old enough for Frank to consider him an old fogy. I hoped he would be able to address the issue so that Frankie wouldn't shut down and start overeating even more.

During his initial examination, Dr. Rucker took my son's vitals, including his blood pressure.

While Frankie was dressing, Dr. Rucker took me aside and said, "Look, I can see that Frank's weight is bothering you or else you wouldn't be here today. But I need you to promise me that you will *not* make an issue of it to Frank. Promise me you will let Frank do this without pressure."

I wasn't sure I understood. Didn't my son need my help? Didn't he want me to intervene and, like always, make everything bad right?

Of course, I'm the first to admit I love Frank unconditionally, warts and all—fat or skinny, short and tall. Maternal love is blind. I knew without reservation that what Frank looked like on the outside had nothing to do with who he was on the inside. I would love him regardless. But his increasing size was starting to scare me.

Then the good doctor dropped the bomb: "Frank needs to lose this weight on his own, when *he's* ready. Any intervention before that will surely give him a reason to develop an eating disorder."

The doctor's words stunned me—perhaps because what he said was exactly what I had feared most. An eating disorder was the last thing Frank needed. That would make the task of losing weight an even higher hurdle to get over, for both of us.

I had seen the after-school movies, read all the warning signs and bleak prognoses in publications like *Parents' Magazine* and *McCall's*. But I hadn't seen much written about teenage boys and eating disorders. The mere thought of Frank's wrestling—battling—this for the rest of his life terrified me.

Maybe Dr. Rucker was right. I needed to give Frank some space.

I needed to take a step backwards. If Frank needed my help, if he wanted my help, *he* would have to ask for it, when, as Dr. Rucker suggested, *he* was ready.

Unfortunately this was no easy feat, especially when Rucker announced that "Frank has dangerously high blood pressure." Dangerously high?

I started to tremble and got palpitations just hearing the words. I don't have to tell you how upset, how preoccupied, I was on our drive home. It continued all through dinner that night and even more so at bedtime and for the entire next day. I had to force myself to stay quiet.

Much to my delight Dr. Rucker's reverse psychology worked its magic.

The next night at dinner Frank announced that he wanted to start a diet. "Maybe you could sign me up for Weight Watchers," he told me. He had seen the commercials, and he went online and read some of the testimonials about the positive results of the program on the Weight Watchers Web page. He even heard his Aunt Angel brag about her special menus and recent fifteen-pound weight loss.

Frank and I spoke in private for nearly an hour. And we began to plan his program almost immediately. He knew he was going to lose the weight, but he didn't know what it was going to take. He asked me to call Weight Watchers and order the necessary reading materials and special menus which would probably be a good place to start.

I'm sure Frank's surge in motivation had something to do with the genesis of *Growing Up Gotti*—a reality TV series on A&E that revolves around my being a single mom raising three teenage sons.

We had just reviewed a tape of preliminary footage—dubbed a demo in the biz—and I imagine Frank was quite unhappy with what he saw of himself—his ballooning image, especially since all of us know that the camera can be cruel and add an additional ten to fifteen pounds on all of us.

I imagine Frank realized he would be seen and watched by his peers, not to mention untold hundreds of strangers—including a few pretty young girls—fans. No doubt he wanted to look his absolute best rather than be made fun of as the fat kid brother. I'm sure he saw that coming.

Frank's eagerness to get started wouldn't allow him to wait for the Weight Watchers material to arrive. That night at dinner he ate half of what was usually on his plate, no seconds, no desserts.

From that time on, Frank cut down, nearly cut out altogether, the bread, sweets, and other fattening treats he normally consumed. He made a conscious effort to change his daily eating habits and to lose weight. And I knew he was serious: he wasn't eating ice cream!

The pounds came off like water. It looked like thirty pounds in the first month!

Frank was astounded at his own progress. As for me, I had never been prouder. Sure, over the years, Frank had given me plenty of reasons to brag like the time he received a special award at school—from the district—for maintaining First Honors four consecutive years or the time he won MVP in his school's basketball program.

Frank's accolades and impressive academic and behavioral skills were a given. These came naturally to him. But his ability to manage his weight was brand new.

I knew how hard it was for Frank to lose weight. It is incredibly difficult for adults to begin and stick to a winning weight-loss program, and Frank is just a kid. (I know it embarrasses him, but I can't help thinking of him as my baby, my little boy.)

The willpower and discipline my youngest son exercised from the start was astounding, and, with each passing day, he impressed me even more!

Relatives would call to marvel at the "New Frank." Neighbors who had watched him grow up would stop and stare as he got on and off the school bus.

Despite their earlier teasing and jibes, Carmine and John also praised him nearly every day. Even those cruel classmates who had made his life so miserable mentioned how good Frank was looking during gym!

By the time shooting for the first season of *Growing Up Gotti* began, Frankie was looking good! He was on his way. He never lost sight of his objective: to lose weight and get fit.

Everyone who has ever battled obesity or attempted to diet and failed knows just how hard the weight-loss process can be, how great the effort, how intense the concentration that is necessary. It takes *work*. It can be daunting to become suddenly physically active after years of living a sedentary lifestyle. That takes a lot of mental effort—like learning to say no to certain foods, such as sweets and unhealthy items. The discipline necessary is not an easy feat, especially when what you really, really crave is something that will only interrupt your quest to lose weight.

Bur Frank wanted to feel and look good even more than satisfying the occasional sweet tooth or craving. For that, I commend him and praise him. I give my son even more credit than I would ever give myself for accomplishing a similar deed.

To those who don't know all of Frank's truly admirable qualities and character traits, my youngest son is a remarkable, incredibly sensitive, aware, and compassionate young man, and, ironically, Frank's battles with the bulge, in the end, taught *me*—the caretaker, the expected leader, the mother—a few lessons in self-control, discipline, and character enhancement that I could never learn on my own.

—VICTORIA GOTTI

RECIPES FOR SUCCESSFUL WEIGHT LOSS

TASTY FOODS THAT

SATISFY YOUR APPETITE

One of the easiest ways to guarantee that you'll stick to your new healthier diet is to fix your food for yourself . . . or convince your mom or whoever prepares the meals at your house to serve up low-carb, low-fat, low-calorie versions of your favorite foods. That's what has worked for me since I made up my mind get in shape.

Believe it or not, my diet hasn't caused problems with the meals everyone else in my family eats either. Sometimes, when Mom has been tied up at work, she has called home and asked me to start dinner. It doesn't bother me at all to boil the ravioli and fry up a few pieces of breaded chicken cutlets for the others. I simply make a huge salad with a good light dressing and grill up a piece of chicken for myself.

If you don't already know how to cook, now is a good time to learn. Just hang out in the kitchen when your mom is cooking dinner and ask her to show you how to do it. I have a confession: I initially learned how to cook, so I could fix myself something to eat if there was nothing in the fridge. That's part of how I got so fat. Now, I cook so I can control the ingredients that go into my meals in order to keep the weight off.

Here's another bit of advice: You'll be more likely to fix your meals the way you need them if you have the right equipment. Your mom probably has everything you need already. All you have to do is ask.

Kitchen Tools I Find Helpful

Table-top grill such as the George Forman Grill
If you don't have access to this equipment, you can use a grill pan to cook on the stovetop or a roasting pan with a rack to cook under the broiler.

Salad spinner
This will spin the water off your lettuce, so you won't have a puddle in the bottom of your bowl. (You *can* live without one: just blot the water away with paper towels.)

Blender and/or food processor

Shaker or jar with lid

Nonstick skillets and baking/roasting pans

Two- or three-cup glass measuring cups (for measuring liquids)

Set of dry measuring cups

Set of measuring spoons

Two or three cutting boards

Use one for meat, one for fruits and vegetables, and the third for garlic and onions if you desire; preferably not wood. Don't confuse them, or you can cross contaminate the food you're cooking.

Several sharp knives

If you can't have but one or two *good* knives, make sure that you have a seven- and nine-inch chef's utility knives.

Assorted long-handled spoons, spatulas, and forks

Pot holders, dish towels, paper towels, and other cleaning supplies

A variety of food storage containers with tightly fitting lids

Aluminum foil, plastic wrap

I am by no means a chef, but I *do* know my way around the kitchen well enough to make the food I need to stay healthy and fit. Here are some of my favorites. I guarantee that every one of them is simple enough for a beginning cook to prepare.

SAFETY FIRST

Okay, so we know we can get burned if we touch a hot stove or if we pull a kettle of boiling water off the burner onto ourselves. Our moms taught us that before we were old enough to dress ourselves. So what's the big deal about kitchen safety?

Let's just say food poisoning is no joke, and food that is allowed to spoil is a waste, making proper food preparation and storage essential to healthy eating. Here are some habits we can cultivate to ensure that we don't make ourselves sick from our own food . . . and that our mom doesn't find her fridge full of science experiments:

- Wash your hands with soap and water before you handle food.

- If you have cuts or scratches on your hands, make sure it is bandaged.

- Store uncooked poultry, meat, and fish in the coldest (lowest) part of the refrigerator. Remove packaging it comes in from the store, and rewrap loosely in waxed paper or foil to allow air to circulate around it. Cook within one or two days after purchasing.

- Thaw any frozen meat, poultry, or fish in the refrigerator. (Put the frozen raw food in a bowl or on a plate so that it doesn't drip on the shelf below.)

- Clean up food spills—on the counter or floor as well as in the fridge or oven—ASAP to prevent contamination.

- Wash your hands frequently while cooking—especially if you've handled raw meat or poultry. (That's why the experts recommend having separate cutting boards for meat and vegetables. The third board is for smelly things like onions and garlic.)

- Store most fruits and vegetables in the refrigerator, and use within three to seven days. A good rule of thumb: Don't buy fresh foods in bulk. Get what you can use within a few days to avoid lost nutrients and changes in taste.

■ Do not store eggs in the refrigerator door. When you open and close the door, you expose the eggs to extreme changes in temperature, which can cause spoilage.

■ Be sure that milk and cream cartons are tightly closed, so the contents don't absorb the odors from other foods in the fridge.

■ Wash fruits and vegetables before using them. Unless you bought them at a farm stand or pulled them off the plant yourself, it might have been dipped in a nontoxic wax to keep it looking fresh.

■ Even if the sign says those salad greens are "pre-washed," wash them again. You never know where it's been on the way to your table.

■ Store fruits and berries that can be easily bruised in the fridge without washing. Rinse them off when you're ready to serve them.

■ When storing leftovers, put the cooked food in a shallow container, cover tightly, and refrigerate promptly. Warm food is a Petri dish for bacteria. In fact, the bacterial count in unrefrigerated food can double in as little as twenty minutes.

■ Toss anything that smells funky. Bacteria also thrives in meats, poultry, fish, stuffing, gravy, cream sauce as well as cream or custard desserts.

■ Don't count on appearance or smell to tell you if food is fresh. If you can't remember when something was cooked, ditch it. Be smart—

when it doubt, throw it out. Your mom won't mind at all if you prevent a family bout with food poisoning.

■ Never eat raw eggs. Enough said.

■ Store cereals, rice, grains, and beans in air-tight containers in a
cool, dark place.

■ Keep bread wrapped in foil or plastic in a cool, dark place. If the
weather is hot and humid, put it in the fridge to keep it from
molding.

■ Discard any bread, cereal, grain, or beans if you see any mold.

■ Use refrigerated leftovers within a couple of days; otherwise wrap it
tightly in foil or freezer bags and freeze.

■ Reheat leftovers *thoroughly* in the microwave or over a double
boiler. This will retain the taste, color, and vitamin content of your
dish.

I don't mean to scare you; the kitchen doesn't have to be as sterile as an oper-
ating room. All I want to do is remind you to use common sense and take care that
everything you eat fits into your healthy way of eating.

LET'S GET COOKING!

Frankie's Chef's Salad

Since salads have been the mainstay of my diet once I started to lose weight, I'm going to start with my own version of that old diner favorite, chef's salad. It is definitely a one-dish meal and, since it has meat, eggs, and cheese in addition to a variety of vegetables, you're getting a good balance of the nutrients you need for energy.

Equal parts iceberg and romaine lettuce

¼ pound lean turkey slices

¼ pound low-fat Alpine Lace cheese, thinly sliced

¼ pound low sodium deli ham (Boar's Head)

1 grilled skinless chicken breast (half of the breast)

¼ cup cucumber, peeled and sliced

2 medium to small plum tomatoes, cut into pieces

1 hard boiled egg, sliced

Low-fat Italian dressing*

Italian flavored croutons (optional)

Wash and dry lettuce. Tear into bite-sized pieces in a large salad bowl. Set aside.

Layer turkey, cheese, and ham and roll into a tight tube. Secure with a toothpick if necessary. Cut roll into four or five little wheels and set aside.

Add tomato, cucumber, and hard-boiled egg slices to lettuce and cover with half of the salad dressing. Gently toss together to distribute ingredients. Arrange the wheels of meat and cheese around the outside of the bowl and add croutons if desired.

Place thick slices of grilled chicken breast in the center of the assembled salad.

Drizzle remaining salad dressing over top of the chicken. Serves 1 as entrée.

*LOW-FAT SALAD DRESSING

¼ cup balsamic vinegar

¼ cup canola, safflower, or corn oil

Salt and pepper to taste

Shake all ingredients together in a covered jar, or whisk in a bowl until completely blended.

You don't have to eat the same kind of salad every day. In fact, you can make a sensational salad from just about anything. You don't even need a formal recipe—just your imagination. So, I've listed some ideas about how to build a salad.

OTHER WAYS TO BUILD A SALAD

MIXED SALAD GREENS

Mesclun, spinach, romaine, red leaf, Boston, butter—even iceberg—lettuces, torn into bite-sized pieces. For a gourmet touch, add sliced endive leaves, arugula, radiccio, or watercress.

FRESH HERB LEAVES (OPTIONAL)

Basil, tarragon, oregano, thyme, or rosemary

SUGGESTED ADDITIONS:

Cherry or grape tomatoes, cut in half, or quartered plum tomatoes

Sun-dried tomatoes, rehydrated in warm water and drained

Red, white, Spanish, or Vidalia onion, thinly sliced

Scallions (green onions)

Carrots, sliced or shredded, or miniature carrots, halved

Celery, thinly sliced

Cucumbers, peeled and sliced

Radishes

Fresh mushrooms, any variety, sliced

Bell pepper, seeded and sliced, raw or roasted (green, red, yellow—it's your choice)

Fresh corn off the cob (can also use flash-frozen corn niblets)

Summer squash (yellow and/or zucchini)

Sprouts—mung beans or alfalfa

Sweet peas, shelled

Pea pods

Artichoke hearts, water-packed, drained

Black or green olives

Capers

Hard cooked egg

Turkey or chicken, sliced

Lean roast beef or steak, sliced

Deli ham, sliced

Water-packed tuna, drained

Shrimp, boiled and peeled

Crab meat, fresh

Surimi (artificial crab made from fish)

Avocado

Apple, seeded and chopped

Orange or grapefruit sections, fresh or canned, drained

Pears, seeded and chopped

Cheese (cubed or shredded): fresh mozzarella, Swiss, Jarlsberg, Gorgonzola, bleu cheese, smoked Gouda, cheddar—anything you like.

Tofu, cubed

Nuts (roasted): pecans, walnuts, pepitas, pignolis, almonds, cashews—it's your choice

To Build Your Salad:

Wash salad greens and either spin dry or blot with paper towels. Place in your bowl. Use more or less, depending on whether you're making it your entire meal or as a side dish to a serving of grilled meat.

Top with tomatoes, onions, carrots—any of the additions in any combination you choose.

MAIN DISH SUGGESTIONS:

Tomatoes, mushrooms, sliced scallions, carrots, corn, capers, artichoke hearts, pitted black olives, quartered hard-boiled egg, sliced grilled chicken breast, crumbled bleu cheese, and almond slivers.

SIDE DISH SUGGESTIONS:

Tomatoes, onion, cucumber slices, chopped bell pepper, mushrooms.

Experiment until you find combinations that you enjoy.

Toss gently together and top with dressing.

You can use any bottled low-fat, low-salt, low-carbohydrate, or low-calorie salad dressing you like—three to four tablespoons per main dish; one to two per side dish—or you can make your own.

Basic Vinaigrette Dressing

In a ten-ounce bottle or jar with a lid, combine:

> **¾ cup extra virgin olive oil**
>
> **¼ cup white vinegar***
>
> **¼ cup water**
>
> **1 to 2 cloves garlic, crushed and chopped**
>
> **¼ teaspoon salt**
>
> **Pepper, to taste**
>
> **½ teaspoon Dijon mustard**
>
> **¼ to ½ teaspoon dried tarragon**

Shake ingredients together until well blended. It will keep in refrigerator up to four weeks if kept tightly covered.

*For variety, use another type of vinegar—balsamic, apple cider, red wine, white wine, raspberry, champagne—as desired. I recommend experimentation to explore a lot of new tastes.

Spinach Pesto Dressing

2 cups fresh spinach

½ cup fresh basil leaves

1 to 3 cloves garlic, peeled (to taste)

½ cup pignoli nuts or walnuts

2 tablespoons grated Romano or Parmesan cheese

¼ cup lemon juice

Salt and pepper, to taste

½ cup water, as needed

Wash spinach and basil leaves and place in the blender or food processor. Add garlic, nuts, and cheese, with lemon juice and salt and pepper to taste. Pulse blender until ingredients are completely pureed, adding water as needed to give it a creamy consistency.

Toss gently over salad as desired. It will keep up to two weeks if stored tightly covered in the refrigerator.

NOTE: This dressing can also be used as a sauce on grilled chicken or fish, such as salmon.

ABOUT BOTTLED SALAD DRESSINGS

If you've never tried any of these light dressings, start small. Read the ingredients to determine if the product is made with flavors you know you like, then buy the smallest bottle possible. If you find you don't like it, you haven't wasted much money.

Read the labels. Stay away from any dressing that contains hydrogenated oil and saturated fat.

Mandarin Spinach Salad

You don't have to go to a restaurant to enjoy a crispy spinach salad. Mandarin spinach salad is one of my favorite meal-size salads.

3 cups fresh spinach leaves

1 cup cherry tomatoes, halved

1cup radishes, thinly sliced

½ pound fresh mushrooms, sliced

1 cup canned mandarin orange sections, drained; 2 tablespoons reserved

1 cup sliced deli chicken breast

Mandarin Salad Dressing*

Prepare Mandarin salad dressing and set aside.

Wash spinach leaves in a sink filled with cold water to remove all sand and grit. Remove stems, and tear leaves into pieces. Dry on paper towels or in a salad spinner. Place in a large bowl. Prepare other vegetables. Drain mandarin orange slices, reserving two tablespoons of the juice for salad dressing. Slice chicken. Add all ingredients to the salad bowl.

Add one-fourth cup of dressing to salad bowl, toss to mix ingredients, and distribute dressing through salad. Serves two as main dish.

*MANDARIN SALAD DRESSING

2 tablespoons mandarin orange juice

½ cup commercial low-calorie Italian dressing

2 teaspoons reduced-sodium soy sauce

1 tablespoon white vinegar

1 packet Splenda or Equal

1 teaspoon toasted sesame seeds

Fine-ground pepper, to taste

Combine ingredients in a jar. Cover tightly and shake vigorously to mix. Refrigerate at least two hours to allow flavors to blend. Makes about three-quarters of a cup. Store in refrigerator for only up to two weeks.

Pasta with Broccoli Rabe

Pasta with Broccoli Rabe is one of my favorite foods of all time. I guess you could call it Italian comfort food, and, before I got a grip on my eating, I'd eat a couple of bowls of it with my meal, especially when Mom added a pound of sweet Italian sausages to the mix.

If you've never tasted broccoli rabe—pronounced broccoli rob—give it a try. It's not just another kind of broccoli, but its flower does look similar to ordinary broccoli florets. It doesn't taste like regular broccoli though. It has a slightly bitter taste that goes well with garlic and pepper.

½ to 1 pound broccoli rabe

2 to 3 tablespoons vegetable oil

2 to 4 cloves garlic, to taste

½ teaspoon red pepper flakes

Pinch of salt

1 chicken bouillon cube

½ cup hot water

½ cup Parmesan cheese

Boil pasta according to package directions until *al dente*. Drain and place in medium pasta bowl. Cover and keep warm.

In a separate pot, steam broccoli rabe to "wilt" the stems and leaves—about four minutes. The broccoli rabe will reduce in volume. Drain.

In a large skillet, heat vegetable oil over medium heat.

Crush garlic, chop it into small pieces, and place in the oil. Cook until the garlic is opaque. Take care that it does not turn brown or burned. Overcooked garlic is bitter and raw.

Add steamed broccoli rabe to the pan and increase heat to medium high. Stir in crushed red pepper and salt. Toss to mix oil and garlic. Reduce heat and cover. Simmer for ten minutes, stirring occasionally.

Dissolve bouillon cube in half cup hot water, and pour over broccoli rabe. Cover and continue cooking ten minutes longer, until broccoli rabe is soft.

Pour broccoli rabe mixture over pasta. Sprinkle with Parmesan cheese, and toss together. Makes two main-dish servings; four side dish servings.

Lemon Pepper Chicken

Lemon pepper chicken is another favorite dinner dish around our house. If you're not carbohydrate conscious, you can even serve this with rice or over spaghetti. Me? I just have a big salad on the side.

1 2- to 3-pound chicken, cut into pieces

1 teaspoon plus ½ teaspoon salt

2 teaspoons black pepper

Juice of 4 fresh lemons extra or ½ cup bottled lemon juice

1 tablespoon red wine vinegar

¼ cup fresh parsley, chopped

Remove skin and excess fat from chicken. Place in a three-quart soup pot and cover with water. Add one teaspoon of salt in the water. Cover and simmer over medium heat for twenty minutes. Remove chicken, and drain on paper towel. When cool enough to handle, pat dry.

In a small bowl, combine lemon juice, pepper vinegar, and half teaspoon salt. Whisk together.

Place chicken flesh-side down in a roasting pan. Pour three-fourths of the marinade mixture over all. Cover with plastic wrap and refrigerate for a half hour. (If it marinates much longer, the chicken will become too sour.)

Preheat oven to 350 degrees. Bake chicken for forty-five minutes, turning every ten minutes.

Remove chicken pieces and place in remaining marinade. Set aside for another five to ten minutes so that the meat can reabsorb its juices. The fresh lemon juice adds another layer of flavor.

Arrange chicken pieces on serving tray and lightly cover with additional black pepper and chopped parsley. Garnish with lemon slices if desired. Serves four to six.

Chicken Paillard

Chicken Paillard just sounds *gourmet. It's just flattened boneless chicken breast that's cooked in the grill and topped with a simple beefsteak tomato salsa. Mom likes to serve it with an endive salad.*

2 whole boneless, skinless chicken breasts, cut in half

4 fresh beefsteak tomatoes

4 cloves garlic, minced

¼ cup balsamic vinegar

1 tablespoon vegetable oil

Fresh parsley, to taste

Salt and pepper, to taste.

To prepare salsa: Chop tomatoes into small cubes. Set aside.

In a covered jar, place garlic, vinegar, oil, chopped parsley, and salt and pepper to taste. Shake to mix thoroughly. Pour over chopped tomatoes and toss gently to combine. Cover loosely and set aside.

Place chicken breast halves between two sheets of plastic wrap or waxed paper and pound very thin. If you don't have a meat tenderizing "hammer," use the bottom of a small, heavy frying pan.

Preheat tabletop grill or grill pan until hot. Grill flattened chicken breasts for two to three minutes or until browned.

Arrange grilled chicken on the platter and spoon tomato salsa over each piece of chicken. Serves two to four.

Endive Salad

1 medium-size head of endive

2 tablespoons crumbled Gorgonzola or bleu cheese

¼ cup walnut pieces

2 tablespoons extra virgin olive oil

Juice of 1 lemon

Fresh ground black pepper, to taste.

Wash endive and separate into leaves. Pat dry.

Arrange half of the leaves on each of two salad plates. Spoon one tablespoon of crumbled cheese into the center of each endive circle. Top each with half of the chopped walnuts.

Drizzle half of the olive oil and half of the lemon juice over each. Grind fresh pepper over top to taste. Serves two. Recipe can be doubled easily.

Chicken and Pasta Soup

I love soup, especially the homemade kind. I often have a bowl for lunch or as an after school snack.

I'll bet you didn't know that it's been proven that people who eat a cup of soup as an appetizer feel full faster and, consequently, don't feel like overeating.

6 cups water

6 cubes chicken bouillon, or 1 cup canned low-fat, low-sodium chicken broth (If using canned bouillon or broth, reduce amount of water by 1 cup)

2 skinned boneless chicken breasts

1 medium onion, cut into chunks

2 large carrots, peeled and sliced pepper to taste

1 teaspoon dried parsley flakes

2 cups acine di pepe pasta, uncooked (If unavailable, can substitute orzo)*

In soup pot, put water, chicken, bouillon salt, pepper, half of the onion, and all of the carrots and celery. Bring to a slow boil.

After ten to fifteen minutes, when vegetables are fork tender, remove half of the cooked carrots and celery. Place in a blender of food processor with remaining onion and parsley. Pulse and puree until thoroughly blended. Add water or broth if necessary to make smooth. Add this mixture to soup pot. Stir to combine pureed ingredients with larger pieces and broth.

Cover and simmer for one hour.

Remove chicken from soup and allow to cool. Shred with a fork.

In a separate pot, prepare pasta according to package directions until *al dente*. Drain and set aside.

Return shredded chicken to the soup pot and add drained pasta. Stir to combine. Reduce heat and continue to simmer twenty minutes.

To serve, sprinkle with low-fat Parmesan cheese if desired. Serves six as main dish; eight to twelve as first course.

*In the early stages of your diet, when you are strictly monitoring your carbohydrate intake, you can eliminate the pasta from this soup and call it chicken and vegetable soup instead.

Quick Minestrone

When you make it the old-fashioned way, it can take hours to cook up a pot of Minestrone. This quick and easy way, using frozen vegetables and canned tomatoes, comes together in less than an hour, from start to finish. It's a hearty soup with a heavy Italian accent.

2 tablespoons olive oil

1 medium onion, chopped

2 cloves garlic, minced

1 10-ounce package frozen green beans (not French cut)

1 15-ounce can garbanzo beans, drained and rinsed

1 15-ounce can crushed Italian tomatoes

2 cups canned chicken broth, or 2 cups hot water plus 2 chicken bouillon cubes

½ cup shaped pasta, uncooked

2 cups water

1 teaspoon dried oregano

1 teaspoon dried basil

½ teaspoon dried thyme

Salt and pepper, to taste

¼ cup grated Parmesan cheese

Heat oil in a large sauce pan or soup pot over medium-high heat. Add onion and garlic and sauté for five minutes until translucent.

Add green beans and sauté for an additional three minutes.

Add all remaining ingredients, except for Parmesan cheese. Bring to a rolling boil. Cover pot and reduce heat. Simmer over low heat for thirty minutes.

To serve, ladle soup into bowls and top each with Parmesan. Serves four as main dish.

Tomato Ditalini Soup

Ditalini is a tiny, tubular pasta that gives this healthy soup its hearty Italian accent. Tomato Di-talini Soup is easy to make as well as tasty. Another plus: you can make it in less than half an hour. If you can't find ditalini in your supermarket, you can use pastina, another type minia-ture pasta, or orzo, pasta that's shaped like grains of rice.

2 tablespoons olive or canola oil

½ cup green bell pepper, seeds and veins removed, coarsely chopped

½ cup coarsely chopped onion

½ cup cucumber, peeled, seeded, and coarsely chopped

3 large cloves garlic, minced

4 large fresh tomatoes, coarsely chopped

1 can (14 1.2-ounce) whole tomatoes, undrained

1 tablespoon vinegar

2 tablespoons dried oregano

Salt and pepper, to taste

1 ounce uncooked ditalini

Heat oil in a large saucepan. Add green pepper, onion, cucumber, and garlic. Stir until pepper is tender and onion is translucent. Add the tomatoes, vinegar, oregano, salt, and pepper. Bring to a rolling boil. Cover and reduce heat; simmer for fifteen minutes.

If desired, remove from heat and allow to cool. Then pour into a blender or food processor in small batches and pulse until smooth.

Return to a boil and add pasta. Cook uncovered for four to six minutes, until pasta is tender. Add water and stir thoroughly. Serves six.

Chicken Cacciatore

You've probably seen chicken cacciatore on the menu at your neighborhood Italian restaurant. Believe it or not, it's a good diet food—as long as you don't pile it onto a plate of spaghetti or eat a loaf of garlic bread!

1 2- to 4-pound chicken, cut into pieces

3 tablespoons vegetable oil

1 medium green Italian frying peppers, cored, seeded, and sliced lengthwise into ½-inch strips

1 medium red bell pepper, seeded and chopped

1 cup sliced button mushrooms

1 cup diced onion

½ cup red wine vinegar

1 cup hot water

2 chicken bouillon cubes

2 cups crushed plum tomatoes (canned)

Salt and pepper, to taste

½ teaspoon dried oregano

Pinch dried red pepper flakes

Cut chicken into pieces. Remove excess fat and skin.

Heat the oil in a large deep casserole or Dutch oven over medium to high heat. Add chicken, turning frequently, for about ten minutes until well browned. Add peppers, mushrooms, and onions. Sauté for about seven minutes, until vegetables are soft but not browned.

Drain off all excess oil and add red wine vinegar to the pot. Sauté for two minutes.

Dissolve bouillon cubes in hot water and stir in chicken bouillon and crushed tomatoes. Season with salt and pepper to taste. Add oregano and red pepper flakes. Bring to a rolling boil. Lower heat. Simmer uncovered for thirty minutes or until chicken is tender and sauce has thickened slightly. Makes four to six servings.

Shrimp Marinara

Another Italian restaurant favorite is shrimp marinara. It's another one of those main dishes that doesn't need pasta or bread to taste great. Of course, if you're not carbohydrate conscious, serve over fettuccini or thin spaghetti. But not too much!

2 tablespoons olive oil

1 to 3 cloves garlic, finely minced, according to taste

2 cups crushed plum tomatoes

Pinch dried oregano

Salt and pepper, to taste

1 pound large shrimp, peeled and deveined, tails removed

¼ cup all-purpose flour

2 tablespoons vegetable oil

½ tablespoon chopped parsley

Heat olive oil in a large skillet over medium high heat. Add garlic and sauté until translucent—about a minute and a half. Reduce heat to medium and stir in tomatoes, oregano, salt, and pepper and bring to a boil. Reduce heat and simmer over low heat for twenty minutes or until slightly thickened.

Place flour on a plate, and drag the cleaned shrimp through it, making sure that you cover thoroughly on all sides. Shake off excess.

In a separate pan, heat vegetable oil. When oil is very hot, carefully add shrimp and cook for three minutes, turning once, until lightly crusted.

Add cooked shrimp to sauce in the other pan and cook, uncovered, for an additional two to three minutes. Remove from heat and serve. Garnish with parsley. Serves three to four.

Shrimp in Fra Diablo Sauce

Yes, I like shrimp! A lot. Here's a spicy dish I enjoy making almost as much as I like to eat it. You can serve it over rice or not.

1½ pounds large shrimp, peeled, deveined, tails removed

½ cup all-purpose flour

2 to 3 tablespoons olive oil

3 small cloves garlic, peeled

½ cup dry white wine

Pinch dried oregano, to taste

Red pepper flakes, to taste

Salt and black pepper, to taste

2 cups plum tomatoes, crushed

4 fresh basil leaves, torn

Place flour on a plate and drag shrimp through it to coat thoroughly. Dip shrimp in flour, coating thoroughly.

Heat oil in large frying pan over medium to high heat. When oil is hot, add shrimp and sauté for two minutes. Stir in garlic and continue cooking for an additional minute, until garlic is translucent.

Remove shrimp from pan and drain off excess oil; set aside. Cover with foil to keep warm. Leaving the garlic in the pan, spoon off excess oil. Pour wine into skillet and stir to remove crusty bits from the bottom of the pan.

Add oregano, pepper flakes, salt, and pepper. Bring to a boil and cook for three to four minutes. Add tomatoes and simmer for fifteen minutes over low heat.

Return shrimp to the pan and add basil leaves. Cook for three more minutes. Serves three.

Fiery Shrimp Sauté

If you like hot and spicy food and shrimp—like shrimp in chili sauce from a Chinese restaurant—I'm sure this simple main dish will become a favorite. You can adjust the heat in fiery shrimp sauté to suit your family's taste buds. Serve with a big green salad instead of pasta or rice, and you'll have one delicious high protein dinner.

1 tablespoon olive oil

2 cloves garlic, crushed and chopped

1 small onion, finely chopped

1 tablespoon chili powder, or to taste

1 teaspoon salt

½ cup water

24 large shrimps, peeled and deveined

1 tablespoon red pepper flakes, or to taste

1 medium red pepper, seeded and finely chopped

½ cup flat leaf parsley, finely chopped

Juice of one lime

Heat oil in large skillet with lid over medium-high flame. Add garlic and onion and cook until tender. Add chili powder and salt, mix well. Take care that garlic and onion are covered with chili powder and that they are not allowed to burn. Add water and reduce heat. Simmer until slightly thickened.

Drop shrimp into the skillet and toss to cover with thickened liquid. Add red pepper flakes and chopped red pepper. Cover loosely and simmer for approximately five minutes.

When shrimp turn pink, add chopped parsley and toss to mix completely. Remove from heat and add lime juice. Taste sauce and add more chili powder, salt, or red pepper flakes if desired. Serves four.

Broiled Filet of Sole

Seafood is truly a healthy part of any weight-loss program. This broiled filet of sole is a tasty change of pace from the more commonly offered grilled salmon or tuna steak.

2 large pieces filets of lemon sole

2 tablespoons extra virgin olive oil

1½ tablespoon all-purpose flour

¼ cup flavored Italian breadcrumbs

1 tablespoon butter

Salt and pepper, to taste

Pinch sweet paprika

Lemon marinade*

¼ cup chicken broth or ¼ bouillon cube dissolved in ¼ cup hot water

Preheat broiler. Lightly brush each filet with oil and place on a baking sheet. Dust with flour and sprinkle breadcrumbs over top side of each. Dot with butter. Season with salt, pepper, and paprika to taste. Pour chicken broth and lemon marinade over all.

Place under broiler. Broil without turning for four to five minutes, until flaky. Remove from heat and serve. Serves two as main dish or four smaller portions.

LEMON SAUCE MARINADE*

½ cup lemon juice or juice from 1 fresh lemon

½ cup olive oil

½ tablespoon red wine vinegar

1 clove garlic, minced

¼ teaspoon dried oregano

Salt and pepper to taste

Mix thoroughly and set aside.

Pan-Broiled Tuna Steaks

These pan-broiled tuna steaks don't taste the least bit like diet food. In fact, this is a show-off main dish for when you want to impress your parents . . . or a date. All you'll need is a crisp green salad, and you've got a feast. The interesting mix of paprika, nutmeg, sugar substitute, and green and black olives give this delicious dish a sophisticated taste.

4 tuna steaks, about 1-inch thick

1 teaspoon salt

Fresh ground black pepper

½ teaspoon sweet paprika

Pinch of ground nutmeg

1 packet Splenda (no-calorie sweetener)

2 tablespoons extra virgin olive oil

¼ cup pitted black olives, chopped

¼ cup pimiento-stuffed green olives, chopped

2 tablespoons chopped fresh parsley

Rub tuna steaks on all sides with salt, pepper, paprika, nutmeg, and sugar substitute.

Heat olive oil in a heavy skillet until sizzling. Pan broil tuna steaks, about four minutes per side, until fish is flaky. Remove to a heated platter and cover to keep warm.

Add chopped olives to remaining oil in skillet and sauté two to three minutes. Scrape brown bits of fish from the bottom of the skillet as you stir olives.

To serve, spoon olives over pan-broiled tuna steaks. Serves four to six.

Baked Salmon in Savory Tomato Sauce

Salmon steaks are another mainstay of a healthy weight-loss diet because they are rich in Omega-3 fat. A variation from the simple grilled fish, this oven-baked, main dish features a savory tomato sauce. Serve with steamed broccoli, steamed green beans, or baked zucchini if desired, or just add a simple salad with a light vinaigrette dressing.

4 salmon steaks, ½ to ¾ inch thick

½ cup flour seasoned with salt and pepper

3 tablespoons olive oil

½ cup finely chopped onion

2 cups chopped celery

¼ cup green bell pepper, seeded and chopped

2 cups canned crushed tomatoes

1 tablespoon Worcestershire sauce

1 tablespoon catsup

1 teaspoon chili powder

Juice of 2 lemons

2 small bay leaves

1 clove garlic, minced

½ teaspoon salt

¼ teaspoon red pepper flakes

Preheat oven to 350 degrees. Dust salmon steaks with seasoned flour and place in a backing dish. Cover with lid or foil and set aside.

In a three-quart saucepan, heat oil and simmer chopped onion, celery, and bell pepper over medium heat for about ten minutes. Add fresh tomatoes, Worcestershire sauce, catsup, chili power, lemon juice, bay leaves, garlic, salt, and red pepper. Cover and continue cooking over low heat, about fifteen minutes, until celery is tender. If desired, process tomato sauce mixture in a blender or strain through a sieve to remove any thick pieces of vegetables.

Pour sauce over salmon steaks. Bake for twelve to fifteen minutes, until fish is flaky. Baste frequently. Serves four to six.

Scallop Kabobs

Scallop kabobs are an especially quick and easy lunch dish that you can cook up on your back-yard grill, in a grill pan, or even on your counter-top grill.

Sea scallops, about 2 pounds—4 to 6 scallops per person

1 small bag miniature "baby" carrots

6 to 8 miniature or pearl onions

1 pint red or yellow cherry or grape tomatoes

1 red bell pepper, seeded and cut into two-inch strips

1 green bell pepper, seeded and cut into two-inch strips

4 large stalks celery, cut into one-inch chunks

MARINADE:

¼ cup olive oil

Juice of 2 lemons

2 cloves garlic, finely chopped

2 teaspoons grated fresh ginger

Salt and pepper, to taste

Combine marinade ingredients in a glass bowl. Marinate scallops in this liquid for at least thirty minutes but no longer than two hours.

Wash and prepare vegetables.

Arrange kabobs on skewers, alternating vegetables and scallops in an attractive order—two to three scallops per skewer.

Grill until scallops are lightly golden and vegetables are tender. Serving size: two to three kabobs per person as main dish. (This also makes a good appetizer for dinner parties.)

NOTE: Don't like scallops? You can use medium to large shrimps or cut chicken cutlets into one-inch cubes.

Bombay Baked Chicken

Bombay baked chicken is one of those exotic-sounding dishes that's so simple to make an amateur cook like me can turn it into a feast. Serve it over a half cup of hot, cooked brown rice once you've lost the bulk of your weight and have settled into a maintenance routing.

¼ cup sliced green onions

2 tablespoons chopped fresh parsley

1 teaspoon to 1 tablespoon curry powder, to taste

1 teaspoon fresh lemon juice

1 6-ounce container plain low-fat yogurt

Salt and pepper, to taste

4 boneless, skinless chicken breast halves

In a 2-quart casserole, combine green onions, fresh parsley, curry powder, lemon juice, and yogurt.

Season chicken breasts with salt and pepper and place in mixture of yogurt and spices. Cover loosely with plastic wrap and place in the refrigerator for at least an hour.

Preheat oven to 250 degrees. Put chicken breasts on a rack placed in a foil-lined roasting pan. Bake for ten minutes then turn and baste chicken with yogurt mixture. Continue cooking for an additional fifteen to twenty minutes, until chicken is cooked through. Serves four.

Chicken with Artichokes

Chicken with artichokes is a simple-to-make main dish that's good for the diet. Boneless, skinless chicken breasts is considered a very lean meat, making this a low-fat, low-calorie, and low-carbohydrate main dish.

> **2 whole boneless, skinless chicken breasts, halved**
>
> **¼ teaspoon salt**
>
> **¼ teaspoon pepper**
>
> **2 teaspoons olive oil**
>
> **Juice of 1 lemon**
>
> **¼ cup chicken broth**
>
> **1 15-ounce can artichoke hearts, drained and cut in half**
>
> **1 teaspoon dried tarragon**

Sprinkle salt and pepper over chicken on all sides.

Heat oil in a heavy nonstick skillet. Sauté chicken breasts on both sides, about four minutes per side. Remove from the skillet and set aside.

Add broth and stir to scrape up browned bits of chicken from the bottom. Reduce heat to medium and add artichoke halves. Return chicken breasts to skillet. Cook for another five minutes. Serves four.

Austrian Pork Chops

This is a special occasion main dish that nobody will believe is part of a healthy weight-loss plan. Believe it or not, pork is a very lean meat that can be flavored with a variety of spices. You can serve egg noodles or rice to anyone who isn't watching their carbohydrate consumption. Serve a crisp salad or steamed broccoli on the side.

4 lean pork chops, ½-inch thick

3 large onions

2 teaspoon dried dill weed

1 tablespoon caraway seed

1 teaspoon sweet paprika

1 pint low-fat or fat free sour cream

Salt and pepper, to taste

Vegetable cooking spray

Chopped fresh parsley, to garnish

In medium mixing bowl, slice onions and cover with water. Add spices and set aside.

Trim excess fat from chops and sprinkle lightly with salt and pepper on all sides. Spray the bottom of a nonstick skillet with cooking spray (Pam) and quickly brown over high heat. Remove chops and place in baking pan. Remove onions and spices from water and place over chops.

Cover with foil and bake at 325 degrees in oven for one hour or until onions are falling apart. Remove chops, cover and set aside. Add sour cream to pan. Stir until blended with onions. Spoon two tablespoons of sauce over each chop and garnish with parsley. Serves four.

Roasted Pork Tenderloin

Roasted Pork Tenderloin is everything I am looking for in something to cook for my diet: It's high in protein and low in fat; it's simple to prepare, and the leftovers are great for jazzing up a bowl of salad. (And my brothers can have their sandwiches.) Serve it with a side salad and something simple—like steamed broccoli, sautéed broccoli rabe, hot spiced applesauce, or corn on the cob. You also might want to roast new potatoes or acorn squash. Experiment with taste combinations. You may be surprised at the vegetables you'll enjoy.

2½ pounds pork tenderloin

1 tablespoon olive oil

Coarse salt to taste

Fresh ground pepper to taste

1 to 2 tablespoon dried sliced garlic

1 to 2 tablespoons dried rosemary

Preheat oven to 350 degrees. Line a roasting pan with aluminum foil, folding up the sides to keep drippings from spreading.

Wash tenderloin and pat dry with a paper towel. Trim off extra fat. Prick with a fork several times on all sides. Place in the center of the foil-lined pan and brush all over with olive oil. Sprinkle coarse salt, coarse-ground pepper, dried garlic slices, and dried rosemary leaves over the top.

If you are also roasting potatoes or some other root vegetable, place on the bottom of the pan around the meat. Drizzle with oil and season with salt and pepper as desired.

Place in the center of the oven and roast, uncovered, for an hour and a half (figure roughly thirty minutes per pound). Remove from oven and cover loosely with foil. Allow meat to rest for twenty minutes to reabsorb juices. Serves six to eight.

Roasted Acorn Squash

3 to 4 acorn squash

Water

Liquid butter-flavored margarine

Fresh-ground nutmeg

Cut squashes in half and scrape out seeds. Place them cut-side down in a roasting pan and pour about half inch of water into the pan—enough to come about a half inch up the sides of your squash but not enough to cover the squash halves. Place in the oven with the pork and cook until tender.

Remove from the water and place cut side up on paper towel to dry. To serve, give the top of each squash half two to three squirts with the liquid butter. Grate a bit of fresh nutmeg on top. Allow one-half squash per person.

Herb and Mustard Rub
(For chicken, pork, or beef)

Who said dieting had to be a sentence to a lifetime of plain, tasteless food? Keep mealtime interesting and add some variety to your grilled chicken breasts, chops, and steak with this tasty wet rub of herbs and Dijon mustard.

  1 tablespoon olive oil

  ½ teaspoon salt

  1 teaspoon Dijon mustard

  ½ teaspoon dried oregano

  ½ teaspoon dried rosemary

  ½ teaspoon dried thyme

  1 teaspoon balsamic vinegar

Stir ingredients together until completely mixed. Cover and set aside for thirty minutes so that flavors can blend.

Trim all skin and excess fat from the meat or poultry you are cooking.

Preheat tabletop grill or bring grill pan or oven to high heat.

Brush wet rub on all sides of your meat and place on grill when it reaches the proper temperature. Cook for two to five minutes per side or until cooked to desired degree of doneness.

Makes enough wet rub for four to six pieces of meat or a whole chicken or turkey breast. Will keep up to a week tightly covered and in the fridge if it does not become contaminated with raw meat juices.

Spiced Apple Sauce

For breakfast, as a side dish to chicken or chops or as a dessert, spiced applesauce is quick, easy, and very good.

1 23-ounce jar unsweetened applesauce

¼ teaspoon cinnamon

¼ teaspoon nutmeg (freshly grated if possible)

Ground cloves, to taste (optional)

1 teaspoon Splenda or Equal

In a one-quart saucepan, stir ingredients together over low heat. Cover and simmer until it begins to bubble.

Can serve hot or cold. Makes five one-half-cup servings.

NOTE: If you're having this dish for dessert, add a tablespoon of low-fat whipped topping or low-fat vanilla-flavored yogurt on top

Pesto Crostini

Pesto crostini is a delicious, quick lunch, appetizer, or special party snack that is high in vitamins and taste.

3 cups fresh basil leaves

⅓ cup low-calorie Italian vinaigrette dressing

⅓ cup grated Parmesan cheese, plus ¼ cup

32 baguette slices (¼-inch thick), toasted

1 8-ounce package reduced fat cream cheese

Wash and dry basil leaves and place in food processor or blender container with vinaigrette and one-third cup Parmesan cheese in food processor or blender container; cover. And process until well blended.

Cover toasted baguette slices evenly with cream cheese spread, then with pesto mixture. Sprinkle evenly with remaining one-fourth cup Parmesan cheese.

Makes sixteen slices. Serve two slices as lunch or appetizer; one slice per snack serving.

Mom's Low-Fat Linguini with White Clam Sauce

One of my favorite foods ever is Linguini in White Clam Sauce. Here's how my Mom makes it.

12 ounces linguini

2 tablespoons olive oil

1½ pounds Little Neck clams (scrubbed)

3 garlic cloves, minced

¼ cup dry white wine

1 cup clam juice

3 tablespoons fresh parsley, chopped

Salt and pepper to taste

In a large pot, boil water for pasta and prepare according to package instructions.

In a large skillet, heat the olive oil over medium heat. Add garlic and sauté for two to three minutes until the garlic is translucent. Add clams, clam juice and white wine. Cover. Bring to a boil, reduce heat, and continue cooking until clams open.

Drain pasta and stir linguini and chopped fresh parsley into the pan with the clam mixture. Season with salt and pepper to taste. Serve on a platter. Serves four to six.

Red Snapper with Lemon

Seafood is always a good choice when you're watching your weight. Here's an easy-to-make en-trée that Mom often cooks for company.

4 tablespoons olive oil

3 garlic cloves, chopped

⅓ cup white wine

2 tablespoons oregano, chopped

3½ tablespoons lemon juice

4 red snapper filets, 4 to 6 ounces each

3 tablespoons parsley, chopped

2 lemons, sliced

Salt and pepper to taste

Preheat oven to 400 degrees.

Prepare marinade by combining olive oil, garlic, oregano, white wine, and lemon juice in a medium bowl. Place snapper fillets in a shallow baking dish large enough to arrange filets in a single layer. Pour marinade over fish. Add salt and pepper. Bake twenty minutes until fish is flaky.

Remove from oven and garnish with fresh parsley and lemon slices. Serves four.

Terrific Turkey Burger

Did you think I'd give up burgers? Not on your life. Here's the recipe for Turkey Burgers that Mom concocted. You need veggies in these to keep the burgers moist—turkey burgers can get dried out real easy.

1 pound ground turkey

¼ cup onion, chopped

¼ cup mushrooms, chopped

2 tablespoons Italian flavored breadcrumbs

1 egg white

2 fresh whole wheat hamburger buns

In a mixing bowl, knead turkey, onion, mushrooms, breadcrumbs, and egg together. Shape into four patties.

Broil in oven or on table-top grill until cooked to your liking.

Serve on toasted buns with lettuce and tomato and whatever condiment you desire. Makes four burgers. You can even leave off the buns and save the carbs!

Peppers and Eggs, Frankie Style

Another favorite breakfast of mine is peppers and eggs, but this dish is made with egg whites or egg substitute to lower cholesterol and calories. It can be served over whole wheat Italian bread.

1 pint container Egg Beaters or other egg substitute

1 pat of butter or I Can't Believe It's Not Butter

1 small white onion, chopped

2 green bell peppers

1 yellow pepper

1 small loaf whole wheat Italian bread (Cut off ends)

Peel and slice onion into rings. Wash peppers and remove stems, seeds, and veins. Cut into 1-inch strips.

Heat margarine in skillet. Add peppers and onion to skillet. Cover and cook for ten minutes over low flame until tender.

Add Egg Beaters and heat until mixture thickens, tipping skillet until top mixture is cooked through.

Slice whole wheat Italian bread lengthwise and then cut in half. Divide peppers and egg mixture on each piece, open face style. Add salt and pepper (and ketchup if you like) and enjoy. Serves four.

Frankie's Sautéed Steak and Vegetables Teriyaki Style

I could eat this great steak and vegetable dish three nights a week!

12 ounces skirt steak, sliced

2 bell peppers

1 red pepper

1 large white onion

2 tablespoons olive oil

¼ cup teriyaki sauce

2 cups brown rice, cooked

Heat oil in skillet over medium heat. Brown skirt steak slices under a minute each side.

Peel and slice onion. Add to steak and stir to combine. Slice tops off peppers and remove all seeds and veins. Cut lengthwise into one-inch slices. Add to mixture. Add teriyaki sauce. Cook over medium heat for six to eight minutes. Be careful that you don't overcook the peppers, or they will turn to mush. Serve mixture over rice. Serves four.

Rappin' Tuna Wrap

Who doesn't like a tuna salad sandwich? Of course all that bread and mayonnaise don't quite fit in with my weight loss plan, so I was glad to learn of this healthy alternative—a tasty wrap sandwich—wrapped in lettuce leaves.

1 6-ounce can water packed white tuna

½ small red onion, finely chopped (about 2 tablespoons)

1 celery stalk, finely chopped

2 leaves fresh basil, finely chopped (optional)

1½ to 2 tablespoons pickle relish

1 tablespoon light mayonnaise

1 tablespoon Balsamic vinegar

6 large romaine lettuce leaves

Coarse-ground black pepper, to taste

Thoroughly drain tuna and flake with a fork. Add red onion, celery, fresh basil, and pickle relish. Stir to combine. In a small bowl, blend mayonnaise and Balsamic vinegar. Pour over tuna mixture and toss to combine. Season with pepper to taste.

TO MAKE SANDWICH:
Spread lettuce leaves on a cutting board and remove coarse stems. Overlap the wide ends of two leaves and spoon one-third of the tuna salad mixture in the center of each. Lift sides around the salad and roll up from one end to form a bundle. Stick a toothpick in it until you're ready to eat. Makes three sandwiches, one per person.

NOTE: You can also serve a scoop of this tuna salad mixture onto a bed of mixed greens or cut a ripe tomato into quarters and spoon the tuna into the middle. You can also substitute shredded grilled chicken for tuna, and even add switch paprika with the balsamic vinegar for a great chicken salad.

Ham and Cheese Tortilla Wrap

If making a lettuce wrap isn't to your liking and you still want to cut down on the bread in your diet, you might want to reach for a corn tortilla. This ham-and-cheese has a Mexican accent I think you'll like.

1 seven-inch corn tortilla

2 to 3 slices deli ham

¼ cup shredded low fat jack or low fat cheddar cheese

2 tablespoons bottled salsa

Heat a dry nonstick pan over medium flame. Place the corn tortilla into the pan and warm on both sides—about fifteen seconds per side.

Place ham and cheese in the middle of the tortilla and top with salsa.

Bring sides up and over the stuffing and roll into a bundle. If desired, return tortilla roll to the pan to melt the cheese. You can also heat in the microwave for 15 seconds. Makes one sandwich.

Hot Turkey Pita Pockets

Want a white bread alternative? Try whole wheat pita pockets. Buy the small ones—the ones the size of a saucer—instead of the hubcap-sized breads and you'll be sure you're not carb loading on your sandwich.

¾ cup low-fat plain yogurt

½ cucumber, peeled, seeded, and chopped

¼ cup chopped onion

1½ cups white-meat turkey, cubed or shredded

1 tablespoon olive oil

¼ teaspoon garlic powder

6 small whole wheat pita pockets

2 cups mixed salad greens

Salt and pepper, to taste

In a blender, combine yogurt, cucumber, and onion. Set aside.

In a skillet, heat the oil and add garlic powder. Add leftover turkey and heat over low heat until warm through.

Cut ½ inch across the top of the pita pocket and fill with hot turkey and salad greens. Top with yogurt-cucumber sauce. Serve immediately. Makes six small sandwiches, one per person.

Chicken Fajitas with Homemade Salsa

If you're going to make fajitas, sometimes that grocery store salsa just doesn't cut it. With this simple-to-make homemade tomato salsa, you can make great tasting fajitas, and it can give an ordinary salad a Mexican flavor.

6 medium ripe tomatoes, seeded and chopped

1 medium yellow onion, finely chopped

1 clove garlic, crushed and chopped

2 tablespoons fresh parsley, chopped

1 teaspoon jalapeno pepper, seeded and chopped (optional)

1 teaspoon honey

¼ cup red wine vinegar

Combine tomatoes, onion, garlic, and parsley in a medium glass or ceramic bowl. Stir in honey and vinegar.

Cover and refrigerate until ready to use. It should keep for up to two weeks.

Makes approximately two cups.

TO MAKE FAJITAS:

Heat a nonstick pan over high heat. Toast a corn tortilla in the pan on both sides until soft. Place a small amount of chopped lettuce on the tortilla and top with four or five thin strips of grilled chicken. Spoon salsa on top. Fold sides of tortilla over chicken and roll into a bundle. Enjoy!

Pita Pizza

Who doesn't love pizza? I do, but I don't want to have all the fat and calories that comes with a slice from the local pizza place. Try using a whole wheat pita for the usual yeasty crust and part-skim or skim mozzarella instead of the whole milk variety. You can cut down on a lot of calories and fat grams.

4 6-inch whole wheat pita pockets

½ cup tomato sauce

1 teaspoon dried oregano, crushed

1 teaspoon dried basil, crushed

2 cups part-skim or skim mozzarella cheese, shredded

Olive oil

Dash garlic powder

Place pita pockets on a baking sheet and brush tops of each with olive oil.

In a bowl, combine tomato sauce, oregano, basil, and garlic powder. Set aside.

Spoon a tablespoon of the tomato sauce mixture into the center of each pita and spread, leaving a quarter-inch border on each.

Top with shredded cheese.

Place under the broiler until cheese melts, one to two minutes. Serves four.

Mixed Berries and Cream

Before I started my diet, I wouldn't have given this dessert a second look. It's not chocolate; it's not ice cream—you get the picture. Now it's something I really enjoy, and I can always find the ingredients in the kitchen when I get the urge to eat something sweet. Of course, fresh juice and berries are best, but frozen berries will taste just as good.

4 tablespoons orange juice

½ teaspoon fresh orange rind

1 tablespoon Splenda

1 cup fresh strawberries

1 cup fresh blueberries

1 cup fresh raspberries or blackberries

Whipped cream or frozen whipped topping

Combine orange juice, orange zest, and Splenda, stirring until Splenda is dissolved, in a large glass bowl.

If using fresh fruit, remove stems from strawberries, wash and cut into halves. If using frozen strawberries, cut in half.

Wash blueberries, raspberries, or blackberries and shake out excess water.

Put berries in the bowl with the orange and sugar mixture; toss gently to mix and spoon into six dessert bowls.

Top each with two tablespoons whipped cream or whipped cream topping. (Yes, you can have whipped cream . . . just not a whole can of Reddi-Whip. It's called portion control.)

Garnish with orange rind curls or mint sprigs if desired. Makes four one-half-cup servings

Mixed Berry Pudding

The same berries and cream can be cooked *to make a luscious pudding. Why not give this variation a try?*

5 tablespoons orange juice

½ teaspoon fresh orange rind

½ cup light cream

1 tablespoon Splenda

1 tablespoon cornstarch

1 cup fresh strawberries

1 cup fresh blueberries

1 cup fresh raspberries or blackberries

Whipped cream or whipped topping (optional)

Combine orange juice, orange zest, light cream, and Splenda, stirring until sugar substitute and *cornstarch* are dissolved in a three-quart saucepan.

Prepare fruit and place in the saucepan. Simmer over medium heat and stir until fruit is soft and juice is slightly thickened and bubbly. Spoon into dessert bowls and allow to cool. If desired, top each with a tablespoon of whipped cream or whipped cream topping. Garnish with orange rind curls or mint sprigs if desired. Makes four one-half-cup servings

Almost Frozen Fruit Bowl

This hot weather dessert—almost frozen fruit bowl—is almost *as good as ice cream. It satisfies my sweet tooth and has that cold feeling so many easy, low-calorie desserts lack.*

3 fresh, ripe peaches, peeled, pitted, and sliced

3 cups hulled strawberries, leave whole unless very large

2 medium oranges, peeled, cut into sections; seeds removed

1 to 2 cups seedless grapes

1 cup raspberries

1 tablespoon sugar

1 teaspoon fresh lemon juice

½ cup fresh orange juice

Toss gently to combine all ingredients. Pour into a two-quart casserole or bowl. Cover loosely with plastic wrap and put in the freezer for thirty minutes or until fruits are *almost* frozen. Serve in bowls. Can garnish with a dollop of vanilla whipped cream. Serves six to eight.

NOTE: If one fruit isn't available, try something else or buy unsweetened flash frozen fruit. Consider adding cubes of watermelon or cantaloupe, pears, or pitted sweet cherries.

Juicy Fruit Cooler

Sometimes you need something sweet and fresh to drink. You can mix these juices and keep them in the fridge for up to a week, if it lasts that long. When you're thirsty, just put a bit into an eight-ounce glass and top with club soda or seltzer water. You can experiment with juices too. What about substituting low-calorie cranberry juice for the pineapple or lime juice for the lemon?

3 cups fresh orange juice

2 cups unsweetened pineapple juice

1 cup fresh grapefruit juice

1 tablespoon fresh lemon juice

¼ teaspoon vanilla extract (optional)

Seltzer or club soda

Mix juices and vanilla extract in a large pitcher or jar with a lid.

To serve, pour one-fourth to one third cup of the juice mixture over ice in an eight-ounce glass. Fill the glass with seltzer. Makes about ten servings.

Berry-Banana Smoothie

A year ago, I would have laughed if anyone offered me a fruit smoothie. Now, it's a favorite hot weather snack treat. It's also a good and quick breakfast dish or an energy-boosting snack.

1 unsweetened frozen strawberries or blueberries*

1 small ripe banana, sliced

¼ cup 1% milk

1 cup vanilla frozen yogurt or low-calorie low-fat vanilla ice cream

Whole strawberry or blueberries to garnish

In a blender, combine first three ingredients and pulse until smooth. And ice cream and blend until smooth.

Pour into a tall glass and garnish with berries if desired. Serves one.

*For variety, you can also make this smoothie with a combination of berries or any other frozen unsweetened fruit, such as peaches.

Chocolate Banana Shake

This smooth shake hits all my taste buds! It's sweet and refreshing.

2 cups skim milk

1 small banana, sliced

1 teaspoon unsweetened cocoa

4 or 5 ice cubes

Place all ingredients in the container of a blender or food processor. Process until frothy—serve immediately. Makes two servings.

Microwave Baked Spiced Apple

Whether you want a sweet treat for an afternoon snack or as a healthy dessert, this Microwave Baked Spiced Apples recipe fits the bill. You'll want to have one apple per person.

1 apple, any variety

1 packet sugar or sugar substitute

1 teaspoon cinnamon*

Wash and core apple. Place on a microwave-safe bowl. Sprinkle sugar and spices into the hole. Cover with wax paper or a paper towel and microwave on high for four minutes. Let stand for two minutes before eating. Serves 1.

*You can add a sprinkle of nutmeg, ground cloves, or both for a slightly spicier taste.

Black Cherry Fluff

I admit it. When I started my diet, I really did miss that milky smooth taste of ice cream. But this recipe cured my Ben & Jerry's blues.

1 package black cherry sugar-free gelatin

½ cup hot water

1 teaspoon fresh lemon juice

2 containers black cherry low-fat yogurt

1 tub low-fat whipped topping

Pour hot water over the gelatin in a large bowl, stirring to make certain it is thoroughly dissolved. Add lemon juice and stir in two containers of yogurt. Once blended, fold into the whipped topping. Whisk to combine and place in a refrigerator dish.

Refrigerate until firm. Makes six to eight servings.

Fresh Berry Ices

You won't miss ice cream at all if you learn to make this fresh berry ice and keep a batch in the freezer. Italian ices have no fat and not too much sugar. Expect the non-dieting members of your family to raid the freezer after they taste it!

**4 cups fresh berries (about 2 pints fresh strawberries;
4 pints raspberries or blueberries)**

¼ cup superfine sugar

½ cup water

Wash and clean the berries. Remove leaves and blemishes from strawberries. Place in a blender and puree until smooth.

Strain pureed berries through a strainer or cheesecloth into a bowl, pushing with the back of a spoon to remove small seeds. Set aside.

In a small saucepan, pour water over the sugar and simmer over medium heat for about five minutes, stirring until the sugar is completely dissolved. When the liquid forms a thin syrup, pour it over the berry puree until it is the consistency of half-and-half.

Taste the mixture and add a bit more sugar if it needs it. Ripe berries won't need a lot of sugar. Be sure you don't add too much, or it will not freeze properly.

Pour the sweetened puree into a ten-inch square pan that is about three inches deep and put it in the freezer for thirty to forty-five minutes, or until it begins to freeze. Remove from the freezer and break it apart with a fork or wisk. Stir until smooth and return to the freezer. Repeat this process every twenty minutes for two hours until the mixture is completely frozen. Keep the pan covered with plastic wrap in the freezer until you're ready to eat it. Serves four.

NOTE: If you have an ice cream maker at home, you can also pour the mixture into the ice cream maker, which will do all the churning for you. It will probably lead to a smoother consistency.

Berries and Cannoli Cream

I'm Italian. And I love cannoli. They are crusty tubular pastries stuffed with a sweet, creamy cheese filling and dusted with powdered sugar. It's hard to steer clear of Italian bakeries, but I do it. This simple Berries and Cannoli Cream dessert (hold the pastry) is a perfect way to satisfy my taste buds.

1 pint sliced strawberries*

2 teaspoons sugar or Splenda

1 12-ounce container low-fat cottage cheese

⅓ cup powdered sugar or Splenda

1 teaspoon pure vanilla extract

1½ grated orange rind

½ ounce (½ square) semisweet chocolate, grated

In a small bowl, toss berries with Splenda. Set aside.

Use a blender or mixer to whip the cottage cheese until it's fluffy. Add Splenda or powdered sugar and vanilla extract. Continue whipping until fluffy. Stir in grated orange rind.

Divide berries into six dessert bowls and top with cheese mixture. Garnish with grated chocolate. Makes six dessert servings.

*You can use blueberries, raspberries, or blackberries, if desired.

GLOSSARY

If this is the first time you're going on a diet or the first time you're getting really serious about getting rid of your extra pounds for good and getting into shape, then some of the terms I used in this book may seem kind of strange to you. So I thought it would be a good idea to include the definitions of any technical or scientific terms. After all, if you don't understand it, you probably won't stick with it!

AEROBIC EXERCISE: According to the American College of Sports Medicine (ACSM), aerobic exercise is "any activity that uses large muscle groups, can be maintained continuously, and is rhythmic in nature." Aerobic exercise increases respiration (breathing) and heart beat and can be done for an extended period of time, as opposed to **anaerobic exercise**, which employs short bursts of energy. See *Anaerobic exercise.*

ANABOLIC STEROIDS: See *Steroids*

ANAEROBIC EXERCISE: The word *anaerobic* means, literally, "without air." There-fore anaerobic exercise is any high-concentration exercise that involves brief bursts of energy followed by periods of rest. These exercises, such as weight training, work groups of muscles but not the heart and lungs. The perfect complement to aerobic exercise, anaerobics increase strength and muscle mass. Examples include weight lift-ing, crunches, wind sprints, and calisthenics.

ANEMIA: This blood condition results from a decrease in the number of red blood cells or a decrease in the protein hemoglobin that is the primary component of red blood cells. It often occurs when you do not have enough iron in your body to man-ufacture hemoglobin or a shortage of Vitamin B_{12}, which affects the production of red blood cells. Common symptoms of anemia are fatigue and loss of energy, pale-ness, shortness of breath, fainting, and heart palpitations.

ANTIOXIDANTS: Foods that are high in Vitamins C and E and Beta-Carotene are known to reduce cell damage. Research also indicates that they can reduce risks of cardiovascular disease, cancer, cataracts, and other diseases. Blueberries are renown for their antioxidant properties, while other sources include citrus fruits, beans, ap-ples, cherries, plums, strawberries and other berries, tomatoes, as well as leafy green vegetables, artichokes, Russet potatoes, and parsley. Vitamin E is found in such foods as wheat germ, nuts, avocados, while beta-carotene comes from deep yellow and or-ange vegetables and fruit.

ANXIETY: This emotional state manifests in a variety of ways, from the butterflies in the pit of your stomach before you take an exam or are walking up to the front door of your new girlfriend's house knowing that you're about to meet her dad for the first time to an absolute, paralyzing fear of unknown origin. Anxiety is normal; chronic anxiety may require therapy and/or medication.

ARTHRITIS: A condition that destroys the protective cartilage in joints, arthritis limits mobility and causes intense pain. There are several types of arthritis, including the most common forms, *osteoarthritis*, which is the degeneration of most frequently used joints and *rheumatoid arthritis*, which is the chronic inflammation of fingers, wrists, elbows, knees, ankles; causing swelling, tenderness, and pain. Obese young people are at risk for arthritis and joint pain.

BLOOD PRESSURE: The simplest explanation of blood pressure is the force or pressure exerted by the heart in pumping blood; the pressure of blood in the arteries. Measured in two areas, the first—systolic pressure—measures the pressure of the blood against the artery walls as the heart contracts, while the second gauges the pressure against artery walls when the heart relaxes between beats—the diastolic pressure. Average blood pressure for adults is 120/80 mm HG, read as one-hundred-twenty over eighty, and less for anyone under eighteen. Blood pressure that is higher than that figure is considered to be too high and can cause serious health problems, including hear attacks and strokes. This condition is called **hypertension.**

BODY MASS INDEX (BMI): This figure is a good indicator of a person's body fat. Using a formula that includes a person's height and weight, gives you a number that is then plotted on a chart. Your doctor can determine where you fit on the chart and come up with the *percentile* you fit. The chart—one for guys and the other for girls in any specific age group—has three lines—fifth, tenth, twenty-fifth, fiftieth, seventy-fifth, ninetieth, and ninety-fifth percentiles. If your BMI falls in the fiftieth percentile, you are close to the average of this population; ninety-fifth percentile says that ninety-five percent of people in your age and gender range weigh less than you, and you are considered obese. Your doctor is equipped to determine your BMI, but if you *must* do it yourself, kidshealth.com explains how: Write down your weight in pounds. Divide your weight by your height in inches. Then multiply this number by 703. The resulting number is your BMI.

CALORIES: A calorie with a small "c" is a unit of energy. Calories with a capital "C" equal one thousand calories (the small "c" kind) and is used to indicate the caloric value in the foods we eat.

CARBOHYDRATES (SIMPLE AND COMPLEX): One of the three main good groups, along with proteins and fats, is carbohydrates. They provide the body with sugar—the body's primary source of energy. Whole grains are the best source of complex carbs, compounds that break up into two or more sugars during digestion. Simple carbohydrates—the sugars—can be found in fruits and vegetables (glucose, fructose, and sucrose) and milk (lactose) as well as in refined foods. Avoid candy, cakes, and cookies, which are full of the simple carbohydrates that come from refined sugars. They are not very nutritious and represent empty calories when dieting.

CHOLESTEROL: This fat related substance found in the blood can build artery-clogging plaque. The two kinds of cholesterol are High Density Lipoprotein (HDL), which protect the blood system, and Low Density Lipoprotein (LDL), which causes clogging. Combined cholesterol levels should be below two-hundred milligrams per deciliter and, for better health, there should be more HDL than LDL in your blood. Cholesterol levels can be reduced by eating less dietary fat, stopping smoking and consumption of alcohol, and eating more dietary fiber. Increased exercise is important too. (See *Triglycerides*)

COCOA BUTTER: Think of cocoa butter as white chocolate without the sugar, milk, and flavoring. The ivory-colored natural fat extracted during the processing of cocoa beans to make chocolate and cocoa powder, cocoa butter can be deodorized (to remove that distinctive chocolate smell) and whipped into a cream, or butter, and used to condition the skin. While it has various cosmetic uses, cocoa butter is used to erase stretch marks that show up after you've lost a lot of weight.

CORONARY ARTERY DISEASE: When the heart and arteries are unable to carry blood throughout your body, you have some form of coronary artery disease. Fatty deposits can clog your arteries. When that happens, the heart muscle is forced to pump harder to push blood into the arteries because the body needs the nutrients and oxygen in the blood to thrive. Once considered a disease of the elderly, coronary artery disease is being diagnosed in young people with more and more frequency as teen obesity becomes so rampant.

CORTICOSTEROIDS: See *Steroids*

DIABETES: This chronic metabolic disorder occurs when the body is unable to produce insulin and properly turn sugars and starches into glucose. The resulting lack of insulin secretion and/or increased cellular resistance to insulin causes elevated blood glucose levels. Damage to the eyes, kidneys, nervous system, and vascular system are common if blood sugar levels are not controlled. Weight loss and exercise can reverse pre-diabetic symptoms and maintain control.

EPIPHYSEAL PLATES: These soft growth plates are located at the ends of the body's "long bones" in the arms and legs to allow for us to grow and mature. When the body has reached its mature height, these plates harden or seal. Injury to these plates, be it "Little League Elbow" caused by overuse or injury to the plates below the knees caused by leg lifts done with excessive weights, can be painful and cause permanent damage. Consequently, weight training must be deferred until a person's body is close to maturity.

FATS: I'm talking about dietary fats, not the fat on our bodies. Technically known as lipids, fats are found in plants (like olives, nuts, and some vegetables) and animals. The body needs fats for energy as well as for growth and repair. Fats also enhance the taste of our food and helps us to feel full. Excess fats are stored in the body as fatty tissue.

FOOD PYRAMID: A graphic designed by the U.S. Department of Agriculture to explain what constitutes a healthy diet. Introduced in 1992, the original food pyramid has been criticized for recommending that people eat meat at every meal and for not distinguishing between whole grain and white breads. An updated food pyramid was introduced in early 2005 with few changes beyond recommending the consumption of less meat. Harvard nutritionists have taken issue with the USDA guidelines and have introduced its "Healthy Eating Pyramid" that puts another spin on the American diet.

HYDROGENATED OILS: Also called hydrogenated fats and trans fats. These are manufactured by a process that adds hydrogen to vegetable oil. That is, a desirable unsaturated fat is changed to a less desirable saturated fat. Found in many prepared foods because they are inexpensive and extend shelf life of food products.

HYPERTENSION: See *Blood Pressure*

LIPIDS: See *Fats*

MINERALS: Your body needs a small but steady supply of minerals to function properly. This includes sodium (salt), potassium, calcium, phosphorous, and magnesium. We need even smaller quantities of other minerals—known as "trace minerals"—like iron, iodine, zinc, selenium, copper, chromium, and fluorine.

MONOUNSATURATED FATS: See *Fats*. Found in vegetables, monounsaturated fats are liquid at room temperature and, like polyunsaturated fats, may be effective in lowering HDL Cholesterol

OBESITY—MORBID OBESITY: Generally speaking, obesity is when your body weight exceeds your "desirable" body weight by more than 20 percent

OMEGA-3 FATTY ACIDS: This beneficial fatty acid is highly polyunsaturated and has been found to decrease triglycerides and may increase HDL cholesterol (that's the good kind). Omega-3 oils, found primarily in deep-water fish, are also known to expand arteries, increase blood flow, and decrease the stickiness of blood platelets, which help keep clots from forming.

POLYUNSATURATED FATS: Also known as polyunsaturated fatty acids, these fats are essential for health and cannot be produced by the body. The three essential fatty acids—linoleic, linolenic, and arachidonic—are vital for healthy blood and circulation and transport fat-soluble vitamins through the bloodstream. Essential fatty acids are found in fish, whole grains, seeds, and beans.

PROTEIN: These chemical compounds contribute to the growth replacement and repair of the body's tissue. While most protein-rich foods come from meats, fish, eggs, and cheese, plant proteins are found in legumes, peas, and beans, as well as in whole grains. Protein enhances taste and provides energy.

SATURATED FATS: See *Fats.* Saturated fats are found, primarily, in animal products like butter, lard, full-fat dairy products, and beef, although they are also in coconut and palm oil. Solid at room temperature, saturated fats should be limited in the diet as they are found to elevate blood-cholesterol levels dramatically.

SHEA BUTTER: Shea—also known as *karité*—is a giant nut found in Africa, where its bark is used in medicines and its edible meat is served as a vegetable and processed to extract a vegetable oil that can be used in cooking, soap making, and skin and hair care products. It's a natural sunscreen and insect repellant, and its butter is used to treat stretch marks resulting from overweight and weight loss. It is also used to treat chapped lips, rough skin, and calluses on your feet. (See *Cocoa butter*).

STEROIDS: This group of hormone-like compounds, both natural and synthetic, includes strong anti-inflammatory drugs known as **corticosteroids** that are used to treat a variety of diseases, such as asthma and various autoimmune disorders, and **anabolic steroids**, which are testosterone or testosterone-like drugs that increase muscular bulk (anabolic activity) and endurance as well as such androgenic activity as secondary sexual characteristics including hair growth. Other negative side effects of some anabolic steroids are mental problems and serious liver and heart damage. Most anabolic steroids are banned from use in the United States.

TRANS FATS: Also called trans fatty acids. See *Fats*.

TRIGLYCERIDES: Like cholesterol, triglycerides are another type of blood fat. Your ideal triglyceride level should be one hundred sixty grams per deciliter or lower. Like cholesterol levels, triglyceride levels can be lowered by adopting a low-fat and high-fiber diet and getting more regular exercise. See *Cholesterol*.

UNSATURATED FATS: See *Polyunsaturated fats*

VITAMINS: These chemicals—usually complex chemicals—are necessary for the growth and function of the body; however, they are not manufactured by the body. Ideally, you should get sufficient vitamins to stay healthy by eating a balanced diet.

ACKNOWLEDGMENTS

Special thanks go to Steve W. Rucker, MD, of Great Neck, NY; Daniel Hamner, MD, Fellow, American College of Sports Medicine; and Jayne Tear, MA/clinical psychology of New York City who specializes in helping people to learn about body management. Without their information and insights, this book would have been a lot skinnier! Big thank yous also go to Sallie Batson, who helped me put my diet and exercise plan down on paper; my editor, Doug Grad, who helped get the book in shape; art director Michelle Ishay and photographer Quentin Bacon, who helped make me look good on camera; and the staffs at both A&E and ReganBooks for their total professionalism. Finally, thanks go to my brothers, for believing in me.